35 Top- Best Diabetic Snacks Recipes

All-Natural Gluten Sugar-Free Snacks and Healthy Snacks Recipes for a Healthy Life

Table of contents

Introduction

"To keep the body in good health is a duty; otherwise, we shall not be able to keep our mind strong and clear."

We are responsible for taking care of our bodies. And this quote by Buddha stresses the importance of it for everyone, irrespective of health conditions. And if you have one, making the best effort to manage it will benefit you as you would have fewer obstacles for your physical and mental health.

When diagnosed with diabetics, we automatically believe that our life is going to alter drastically. But then, this is a faulty assumption. In a diabetic diet, no food groups or ingredients are off-limit. Instead, a moderate amount of every food item is the point emphasized. The key to control diabetics is the proper management of the menu.

Finding healthy diabetic snacks could be slightly tricky. There are certain conditions you need to consider while choosing diabetic meals. They should be low in calories, sugar, and carb and sodium while being high in fiber, fat, and proteins. When we snack on these nutrients, we should be able to advance our health. So that's why we are here with this cookbook. Through this ebook, we aim to put back flavor and choice back to this healthy diet.

In this book, we have 35 simple and easy to make diabetic snacks recipe for you. Step by step, explanations of recipes in a straightforward manner is given. Furthermore, tips are provided wherein substitutions, if possible, are described. What's more, nutritional information is there so that you have the right understanding. Along with these recipes, we have also explained in detail about diabetics, varieties of diabetics, manifestations of diabetics, and rules of nutrition in diabetics so that you have a complete understanding of the disease that will aid you to manage diabetes effectively without much difficulty.

So why are you waiting to buy this book which has a mine of information about diabetes which you can dig in immediately? The recipes are guaranteed to temp you while contributing to the health and well-being.

Varieties of Diabetics & How do they Differ

Before we comprehend what the different types of diabetics are, it is crucial to understand what diabetics as a chronic disease mean. When someone says they have diabetics, it means that either their body is not producing a sufficient amount of insulin or that their body is not using appropriately the insulin provided, or it can be a combination of both.

A diabetic body is not able to pass the sugar from the blood to the cells. Therefore, their body will have higher levels of sugar in the blood. For the human body, glucose is the primary energy source that nourishes your cell. But for the glucose to enter the cell, it requires insulin. Insulin is the hormone accountable for controlling the way blood sugar becomes energy. The shortage of insulin makes the sugar level rise in the blood, which can then cause numerous health problems. So if a person has diabetics, the level of glucose will always tend to be high unless they are taking proper precautions to manage it effectively.

Now that you know what diabetics is, you can proceed to read what are the three types of diabetics. They are:

- Type 1 Diabetics
- Type 2 Diabetics
- Gestational Diabetics

Vis-à-vis how they differ, we need to understand each of them so that we can effectively treat the health concern.

- **Type 1 Diabetics** – The first type of diabetics is an autoimmune condition. When you have type 1 diabetics, the body's immune system mistakenly attacks and destroys the cells in the pancreas, which is responsible for generating insulin. The beta cells in the pancreas are considered erroneously as foreign invaders by the immune system because of which they are unable to create insulin. Diabetics of this nature are permanent, and the reason behind the occurrence is still not known. They can occur either due to environmental or genetic reasons or both.

This type progresses quickly and can cause symptoms like weight loss, irritability, mood changes, or a condition called diabetic ketoacidosis in which you have a high level of sugar with no or little insulin in the body. There isn't a specific age group, but type 1 is more common in children and young adults. It was called juvenile-onset diabetics for this reason since it usually starts during childhood. The symptoms develop fast.

For treating type 1 diabetics, taking insulin is a must as the damage to the pancreas is permanent. They are injected under the skin into the fatty tissue below and taken after monitoring the sugar levels throughout the day.

- **Type 2 Diabetics** – The most prevalent type of diabetics is type 2 diabetics. The origin of this type is insulin resistance. In type 2 diabetics, the body is not able to use insulin properly and efficiently. The amount of insulin is either less than what the body needs or the body cells are resisting it. As the body is not able to use the insulin properly, glucose gets accumulated in the blood, and the blood sugar level rises. Insulin resistance or lack of sensitivity to the hormone occurs mainly in fat, liver, and muscle cells. When there is insulin resistance, the pancreas needs to work overtime to produce insulin. And still, the amount won't be sufficient to keep the glucose level down. As the glucose keeps on rising, the body becomes overexposed to insulin and becomes less responsive to it.

The reasons for type 2 diabetics can be any of the following:
- Genetics
- Overweight & obesity
- Lack of physical exercise

Type 2 diabetes is prevalent in those aged 45 or more. But in the past decade or so, the disease is noticed even in younger generations due to the sedentary lifestyle and eating patterns. The symptoms start occurring over time.

Treating type 2 diabetics is possible through proper diet and physical exercise, along with the usage of medicines.

- **Gestational Diabetics** – This form of diabetics occurs during the time of pregnancy. Insulin blocking hormones are produced during the time. This type usually appears during the middle and last stages of pregnancy. The diabetics generally resolve by itself once the pregnancy is over.

Manifestations of Diabetics

The main symptoms of chronic diabetics are:

- excessive thirst and frequent urination
- blurry vision
- extreme hunger
- slow-healing wounds
- Dry, itchy skin along with dark patches in the fold of underarms and neck skin
- fatigue
- blurry vision
- numbness in hand and feet
- unexplained weight loss

Those who observe the symptoms mentioned above should see the doctor immediately to get treated effectively.

Rules of Nutrition in Diabetics

When you have diabetics, maintaining a healthy lifestyle is vital. Nutrition and physical exercise play an integral role in the treatment of your sugar levels. Having a healthy meal plan and active, fit lifestyle can support you in regulating your blood sugar to your safe levels. Though what you eat is significant, how much you eat and the mealtimes are also fundamental in the treatment. Being more active and making changes to the diet may seem a bit challenging in the initial period.

But once you start with smaller steps, you will soon find that keeping the sugar levels at your targeted levels becomes easy for you to handle. Regulating what you eat and drink, along with physical exercise and medications, makes the process calmer for you.

For many, just the thought of diabetics conveys the worry that you would have to sacrifice your favorite foods. But then it is not valid. You can have your favorite food but in smaller quantities or at a lesser frequency. The only point which you need to consider is that you have to eat from all the food groups and thereby bring in a variety to all. Alongside, always make sure to avoid the following groups through:

- fried foods
- foods rich in saturated fat and trans fat
- foods rich in salt called sodium
- sweets, such as candy and ice cream
- beverages with a high content of sugars

Eating meals at regular times and at the same time every day, along with a moderate quantity, is the only criterion of a healthy diabetic meal plan. The diet aids the insulin that the body has or which it gets through medicines.

To help you have a healthy meal plan, two standard techniques are adopted usually. They are plate method and carbohydrates counting method. You might need to refer to your practitioner before making changes, though.

Plate Method – Through this technique, you can control your meal size. Rather than getting worried about calories consumed, this method lets you know how much and which each food group you need to take in daily. The technique works best for your lunch and dinner.

So take a 9-inch plate. Place non-starchy vegetables on one half of the plate, meat or protein in the next portion, and finally starch and grain in the remaining last quarter. Spoon in few good fats such as nuts and avocado, and you have the complete one.

Carbohydrate counting – In this method, you measure up the number of carbohydrates you take each day from what you eat and drink. The technique, therefore, aids in managing your level of sugar level concerning carbohydrates. The right level of carbohydrates helps in regulating the disease. How much carbs you can take depends on how your diabetics are maintained, how much you exercise, and what medicines you are taking. It varies with each person. Carbohydrates come from starches, fruits, milk, and chocolates. Try to limit the consumption of refined sugars and instead rely more on carbohydrates from fruits, whole grains, etc.

Diabetic meals are open and are rich in nutrients while being low in fat and calories. Diabetics meal plans are suitable for everyone and not just for the patients. Enjoy foods at regular mealtimes in moderate amounts while tracking your diet, and you are on the right path.

When you are physically active, the following benefits accrue:

- reduces blood sugar levels
- aids in sleeping better
- reduces blood pressure
- burns calories which can keep your weight in check
- enhances blood flow
- mood enhancer

Physical activities of even 30 minutes for five days of the week would be great. If you can, you can also aim for more. But then this is the minimum which you should be able to achieve so to aid you in managing diabetics.

Embracing this healthy diabetic plan is the right method to maintain your blood sugar levels.

Rules of Snacks for Diabetics

To aid in keeping your diabetics in check, you need to make sure that you have healthy snacks, which are a combo of fiber, fats, proteins, and carbohydrates. Snacks help in maintaining the sugar levels in check as they aid in reducing the occurrence of sugar spikes. Choosing those that are having less than 200 calories would be an excellent criterion.

High protein snacks are advisable as these diabetic foods can keep you feeling full for a more extended period without any hunger pangs. The sugar level becomes stable. Similarly, selecting foods with a high level of fiber is also great as they aid in reducing the speed of absorption of sugar into the bloodstream while keeping the sugar level in balance. Fibre also reduces cholesterol and maintains bowel health. So make sure to include high protein, high fiber snacks in your diet.

To make the diet more perfect, you can add healthy fats, which are excellent for your heart. They aid in keeping you feel full for a longer time. The only items which should be out of the diet would be fried foods. Snacks made with whole and unprocessed foods that stable sugar levels and which keep you full should be our quest ahead.

According to nutritionists and dietitians, 80% of our snacks need to be healthy, and 20% can be slight indulgences.

They are three types of snacks, which are advisable for diabetic patients, all of which are under 15gm of carbohydrates. They are:

- **Low carbohydrates snacks** – Those food items which do not require the cover of insulin comes under this category. For example, non-starchy vegetables along with dips.
- **Sustaining snacks** – These snacks are a mix of carbohydrates with a protein source or fat source and are ideal for consumption between two meals. For example, cheese with crackers, etc.
- **Fast-acting snacks** – These snacks are advisable to be taken when your blood sugar levels drop down quickly. They have a

higher percentage of carbohydrates but no fat, fiber or protein. Fat, protein, and fiber can slow the absorption of snacks. Example, a tablespoon of honey or sugar or raisin, etc.

A good rule you need to consider while choosing healthy diabetic snacks is not only to look for healthy foods but also to those who are equally tasty and satisfying for you. Smaller bites should always have less than 15gm of carbohydrates. And among carbohydrate foods, always go for vegetables, fruits, legumes, and whole grains instead of carbs from white rice, flour, and sugar.

Be mindful of the dietary choices, and we have the right path head.

Sugar Substitutes

Once diagnosed with diabetics, we automatically assume that we can't have any more sweet dishes or any sweetness in our meals. But then, this assumption is faulty and untrue. With alternative sweeteners, we can consume sweet fares at the bare minimum level.

Artificial sweeteners are low-calorie sweeteners that can avoid sugar spikes in diabetic patients as they do not affect blood sugar levels. But then, all artificial sweeteners are not good and can cause more problems than table sugar. Some of these have more calories and sugar content than the regular sugar and, therefore, should be avoided entirely. For this reason, we should select them after much consideration.

1. **Stevia** – One of the most popular low-calorie sweeteners available in the market is stevia. This natural sweetener is extracted from the Stevia Rebaudiana plant and is 300 times sweeter than regular sugar and sucrose. The main advantage of using this natural sweetener is its low-calorie content. Because of its slightly bitter aftertaste and higher price, many people look out for other similar sweeteners in the market.

2. **Tagatose** – Another form of fructose used widely is tagatose. This sweetener is 90% sweeter than sucrose. Many fruits like orange, pineapple can provide tagatose naturally. Several studies have reported that tagatose can aid in the management of type 2 diabetics because of its low glycemic index. This index is a measuring system that ranks food items based on its capacity to increase a person's blood sugar level. But then, tagatose is more expensive and harder to find in stores.

3. **Sucralose** – This is a low-calorie sweetener made from sucrose. Sucralose or Splenda is widely popular and is the artificial sweetener that is used more. When people are looking for sweeteners for sugar-free baking, Splenda is the first choice as they do not lose their taste at high temperatures.

Glycemic Index Food Chart

An excellent way to regulate the level of glucose in diabetic patients is through the measurement of carbohydrates. The glycemic index food chart is one such useful tool that can aid in the management. In this index, an assigned value is given to every food item based on its ability to raise the sugar level in the body. Foods that have a low glycaemic index can release the sugar slowly into the bloodstream, whereas the ones which have high glycemic index aid with energy recovery after exercise as they release sugar in a fast mode or rapidly.

Now, diabetic patients should look out for food items that have a low glycemic index. The reason behind is that the slow release of glucose in low GI food aid in keeping blood glucose under control. Furthermore, low GI food can also help if you are looking to reduce body weight. To help you further in this process, we are providing a glycemic index chart of 60 common food items. The chart was released in the 'Diabetics care' and was released by the American Diabetics Association.

FOOD	GLYCEMIC INDEX (Glucose= 100)
High-Carbohydrate Foods	
White wheat bread*	75 ± 2
Whole wheat/wholemeal bread	74 ± 2
Specialty grain bread	53 ± 2
Unleavened wheat bread	70 ± 5
Wheat roti	62 ± 3
Chapatti	52 ± 4
Corn tortilla	46 ± 4
White rice, boiled*	73 ± 4
Brown rice, boiled	68 ± 4
Barley	28 ± 2
Sweet corn	52 ± 5
Spaghetti, white	49 ± 2

Spaghetti, whole meal	48 ± 5
Rice noodles†	53 ± 7
Udon noodles	55 ± 7
Couscous†	65 ± 4
Breakfast Cereals	
Cornflakes	81 ± 6
Wheat flake biscuits	69 ± 2
Porridge, rolled oats	55 ± 2
Instant oat porridge	79 ± 3
Rice porridge/congee	78 ± 9
Millet porridge	67 ± 5
Muesli	57 ± 2
Fruit And Fruit Products	
Apple, raw†	36 ± 2
Orange, raw†	43 ± 3
Banana, raw†	51 ± 3
Pineapple, raw	59 ± 8
Mango, raw†	51 ± 5
Watermelon, raw	76 ± 4
Dates, raw	42 ± 4
Peaches, canned†	43 ± 5
Strawberry jam/jelly	49 ± 3
Apple juice	41 ± 2
Orange juice	50 ± 2
Vegetables	
Potato, boiled	78 ± 4
Potato, instant mash	87 ± 3
Potato, french fries	63 ± 5
Carrots, boiled	39 ± 4
Sweet potato, boiled	63 ± 6
Pumpkin, boiled	64 ± 7
Plantain/green banana	55 ± 6
Taro, boiled	53 ± 2

Vegetable soup	48 ± 5
Dairy Products And Alternatives	
Milk, full fat	39 ± 3
Milk, skim	37 ± 4
Ice cream	51 ± 3
Yogurt, fruit	41 ± 2
Soy milk	34 ± 4
Rice milk	86 ± 7
LEGUMES	
Chickpeas	28 ± 9
Kidney beans	24 ± 4
Lentils	32 ± 5
Soya beans	16 ± 1
Snack Products	
Chocolate	40 ± 3
Popcorn	65 ± 5
Potato crisps	56 ± 3
Soft drink/soda	59 ± 3
Rice crackers/crisps	87 ± 2
Sugars	
Fructose	15 ± 4
Sucrose	65 ± 4
Glucose	103 ± 3
Honey	61 ± 3
Data are means ± SEM.	
* Low-GI varieties were also identified.	
† Average of all available data.	

Risk Factors For Diabetics

A recent medical study report done in the United States of America points out that one in every four patients with diabetics do not realize that they have diabetics. Would you like to know whether you are at risk of developing this chronic disease? Then continue reading this article and make suitable healthy changes to prevent it further if you notice any of these factors.

- **Type 1 Diabetics** – This type usually starts occurring during childhood itself. The damage which has happened to the pancreas is permanent, and therefore the person will have to suffer from it throughout their life. Some of these are:
    - ✓ Family History
    - ✓ Pancreatic Diseases
    - ✓ Infection or illness.

- **Type 2 Diabetics** – When there is an occurrence of insulin resistance, there is a high chance of you getting type 2 diabetics. For this, the phenomenon can happen at any time. The factors leading can be:
    - ✓ Obesity
    - ✓ Family History
    - ✓ Sedentary Lifestyle
    - ✓ Pre-diabetics
    - ✓ Insulin resistance

Irrespective of your risk factors, always try to ensure proper care of your body as they are lot of things which you can do.

FAQ, Common Mistakes and How to Avoid them

When you have diabetics, and if you have just started on this journey, you are bound to make some mistakes. So here we are to inform some of the mistakes we have seen around and also the solutions for them so that you don't repeat them.

1. **Not recording sugar level reading** – Once you are on diabetic management, you must register your readings of sugar level continuously based on your history. The recordings will help you as well the medical practitioner to understand situations with much more clarity.
2. **Avoiding carbohydrates altogether** – Though carbohydrates should be limited, it doesn't mean we should eliminate carbohydrates. There are good carbohydrates which you can take in a moderate amount.
3. **Not doing sufficient exercise** – Without physical activity, it would be highly hard to treat diabetics. Physical exercises reduce the level of sugar naturally while making you feel better.

Now regarding diet control. They are indeed few rules about dieting, which you can follow to help you to be on track when you have diabetics and to get the maximum out of each of the meals.

1. **Never stay hungry** – Make sure you are always full after every meal. If not, there is a chance that you would try to fill up by eating unnecessary food items,
2. which may cause unwanted sugar spikes. Alongside this, it may also cause hypoglycemia when you are waiting too long between meals.
3. **Snacks should be less than 200 calories, preferably** – If the number of snacks taken goes abroad, then there is a possibility

of it becoming an extra meal, which is unnecessary while increasing the calorie intake.

4. **Always watch the quantities** – The amount of food you take at every meal should satisfy and make you feel full.

5. **Take clean beverages** – Try to eliminate drinks that have calories and instead go for water or healthy ones like herbal teas or black teas. Similarly, fruit juices can lead to a rise in sugar levels immediately.

6. **Always aim for a combo of three nutrients at every snack** – Every snack can be a combo of carbohydrates, fat, and protein so that they remain full for a more extended period while keeping hunger pangs at bay. On top, their energy levels will also be high.

7. **Have a filling breakfast** – When you start your day with a healthy breakfast, you are set up for healthy eating. Go for a rich source of protein and carbs. This helps you to not crush out later on during the day.

Recipes

Almond Butter Energy Balls

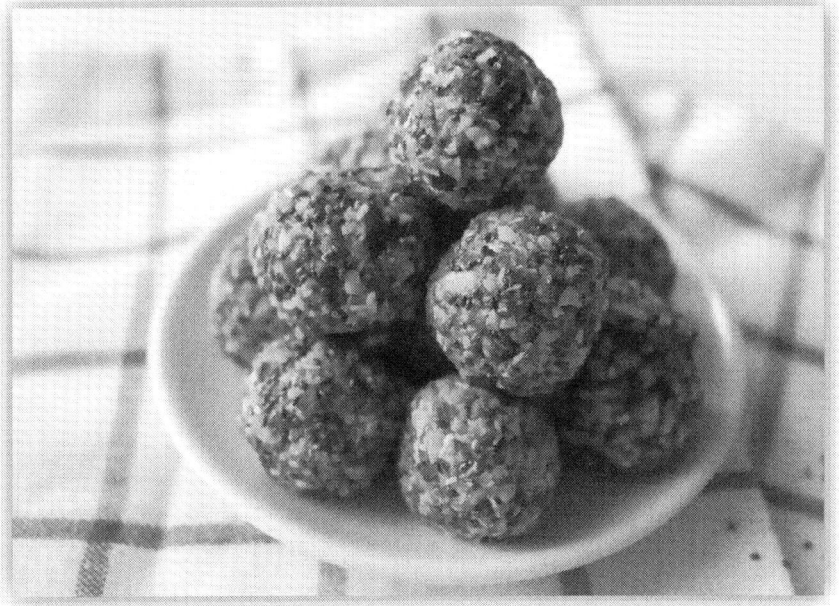

Preparation Time: 20 Minutes
Cooking Time: 0 Minutes
Servings: 17 Balls

Ingredients:

- 2 cups Oats, rolled
- ¼ cup Shredded Coconut, unsweetened
- ½ cup Honey
- ¼ cup Nuts, chopped
- 1 cup Almond Butter

Method of Preparation

- Combine oats, honey, shredded coconut, almond butter, and chopped nuts in a medium-sized bowl.
- Mix the coconut mixture well until you get a smooth dough.
- After that, with the help of 1 tablespoon spoon, make balls out of the dough.
- Store the energy balls in an air-tight container in the refrigerator for five days or in the freezer for three months.

Tip: Instead of nuts, you can also use dried fruits or even chocolate chips if you desire.

Nutritional Information per serving: (2 balls = 1 serving)
- ✓ Calories: 174Kcal
- ✓ Carbohydrates: 16g
- ✓ Proteins: 4g
- ✓ Fat: 9g
- ✓ Sodium: 48mg

Deviled Eggs

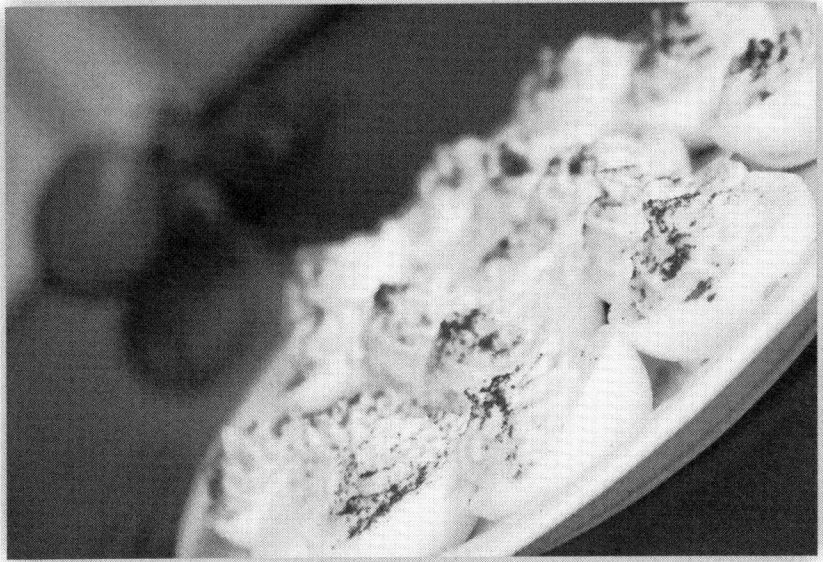

Preparation Time: 10 Minutes
Cooking Time: 30 Minutes
Servings: 12

Ingredients:

- 6 Eggs, preferably farm-raised
- 1 tbsp. Red Pepper, roasted
- ¼ cup Cottage Cheese, low-fat
- 2 tbsp. Chives, fresh & chopped
- 3 tbsp. Ranch Dressing, homemade with less fat
- 2 tsp. Dijon Mustard

Method of Preparation

- To start with, place eggs in a medium-sized saucepan filled with water. Cover with a lid.
- Boil the water over high heat. Remove from heat.
- Keep it aside for 10 to 13 minutes and then drain away the cold water.
- Pour cold water to the pan and set it aside until the eggs are cooled. Drain the water and peel the eggs.
- Now, slice the eggs into two portions lengthwise while removing the egg yolk. Reserve three egg yolks.
- Then, keep the egg whites with the cut side up on a plate and cover it with a plastic wrap.
- Place it in the refrigerator until needed.
- After that, to make the filling, stir cottage cheese, three egg yolks, ranch dressing, and mustard in a food blender and blend for a minute. The mixture should be smooth without any lumps.
- Pour the mixture to a small-sized bowl and add the pimento and chives to it. Mix again.
- Finally, spoon the mixture into the well of the egg whites. Place it in the refrigerator until served.

Tip: Instead of chives, you can also use dill.

Nutritional Information per serving: (1 filled egg half = 1 serving)
- ✓ Calories: 44Kcal
- ✓ Carbohydrates: 1g
- ✓ Proteins: 4g
- ✓ Fat: 3g
- ✓ Sodium: 96mg

Roasted Pumpkin Seeds

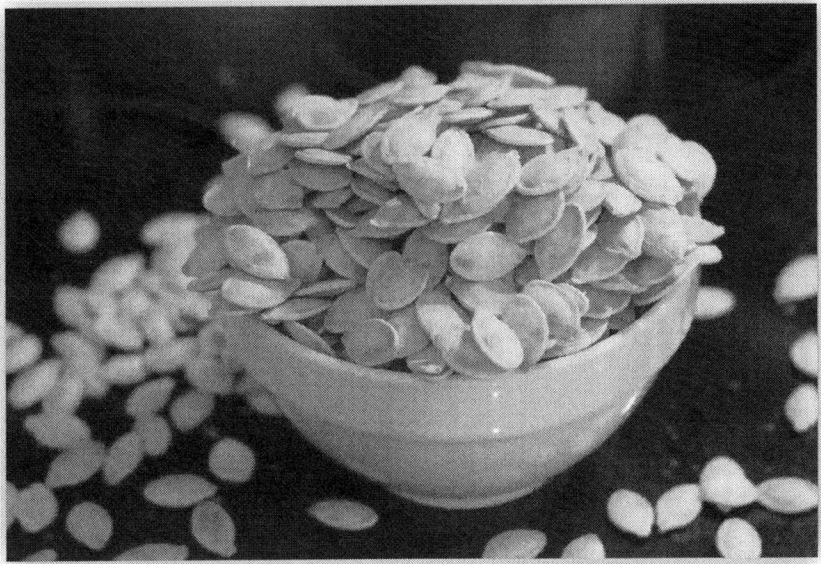

Preparation Time: 10 Minutes
Cooking Time: 45 Minutes + 10 cooling time
Servings: Makes 2 cup

Ingredients:

- 2 cups Pumpkin Seeds, fresh
- ½ tsp. Salt
- 5 tsp. Butter, melted
- ¼ tsp. Cayenne Pepper
- 1 tbsp. Worcestershire Sauce
- ¼ tsp. Garlic Powder
- 1 tsp. Sugar

Method of Preparation

- To start with, preheat the oven to 250 ° C.
- After that, place the pumpkin seeds in a medium-sized mixing bowl along with melted butter and Worcestershire sauce. Combine well.
- Next, stir in all the remaining ingredients to the mixing bowl. Mix again.
- Now, transfer them to a greased baking sheet or pan while leaving ample space between them.
- Then, bake them for 48 to 60 minutes while stirring it occasionally or until they are light brown in color and dry.
- Allow them to cool completely before storing.

Tip: You can use favorite seasoning.

Nutritional Information per serving: (1/4 cup = 1 serving)
- ✓ Calories: 96Kcal
- ✓ Carbohydrates: 9g
- ✓ Proteins: 3g
- ✓ Fat: 6g
- ✓ Sodium: 176mg

Chia Seed Bread

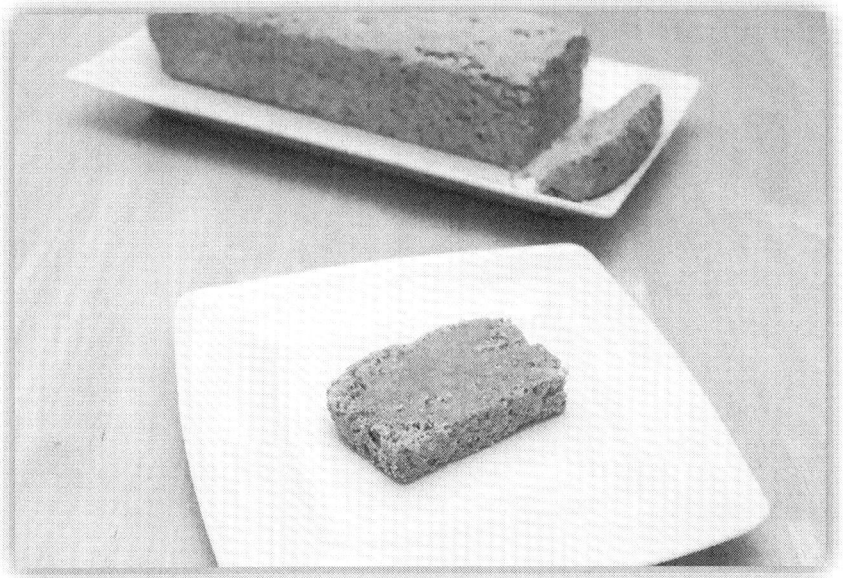

Preparation Time: 20 Minutes
Cooking Time: 45 Minutes
Servings: Makes 1 loaf or 12 slices

Ingredients:

- 1 cup Greek Yoghurt
- 2 tbsp. Coconut Flour
- 1 pinch of Salt
- 3 Eggs, preferably farm-raised
- ½ tbsp. Baking Powder
- 3 tbsp. Chia Seeds
- 1 cup Almonds, grounded
- 3 tbsp. Psyllium Husk Powder

Method of Preparation

- First, combine eggs and Greek yogurt in a large mixing bowl with a beater until you get it smooth.
- After that, stir in the grounded almonds, baking powder, coconut flour, and salt to the bowl. Mix again.
- Next, spoon in the chia seeds and psyllium husk into it.
- Give a good stir so that everything comes together.
- Now, transfer the batter to a greased parchment paper-lined loaf pan.
- Allow the batter to rest for 15 minutes.
- Preheat the oven to 340 ° F.
- Finally, bake them for 40 to 45 minutes or until the bread is lightly browned, and a skewer inserted in the middle portion comes clean.

Tip: You can also add sunflower seeds if needed.

Nutritional Information per serving: (1 to 2 slices = 1 serving)
- ✓ Calories: 107Kcal
- ✓ Carbohydrates: 6.3g
- ✓ Proteins: 7.6g
- ✓ Fat: 6.3g
- ✓ Sodium: 67mg

Tomato Salsa

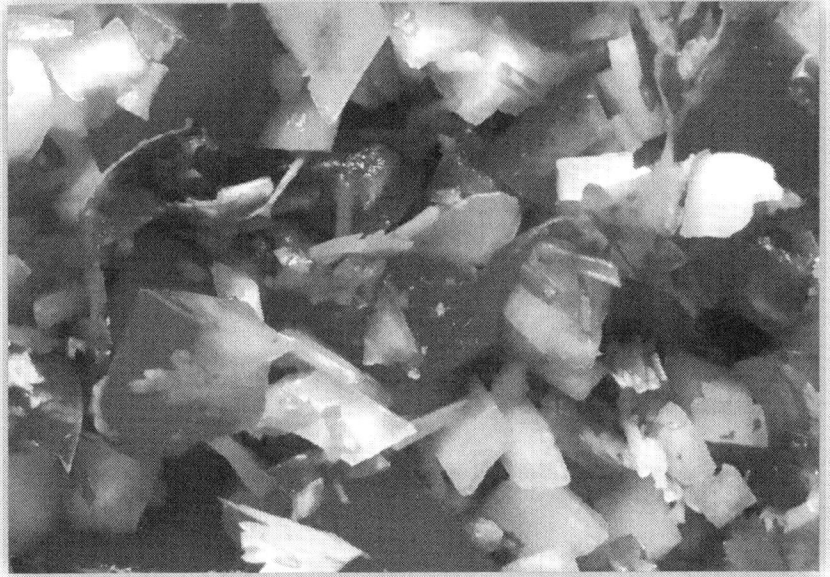

Preparation Time: 10 Minutes
Cooking Time: 20 Minutes
Servings: 12

Ingredients:

- 3 Tomatoes, medium & diced
- 2 tsp. Marjoram, fresh & chopped finely
- 1 Garlic clove, minced
- 2 tbsp. White Onion, chopped finely
- ½ tsp. Kosher Salt
- Pepper, to taste

Method of Preparation

- For making this easy snack, you need to first mash the garlic and salt together.
- After that, mix all the remaining ingredients in a medium-sized mixing bowl along with the garlic paste. Combine.
- Serve and enjoy.

Tip: You can serve this salsa warm or cold.

Nutritional Information per serving: (4 tbsp. = 1 serving)

- ✓ Calories: 5Kcal
- ✓ Carbohydrates: 0g
- ✓ Proteins: 4g
- ✓ Fat: 0g
- ✓ Sodium: 81mg

Sweet Potato Toast

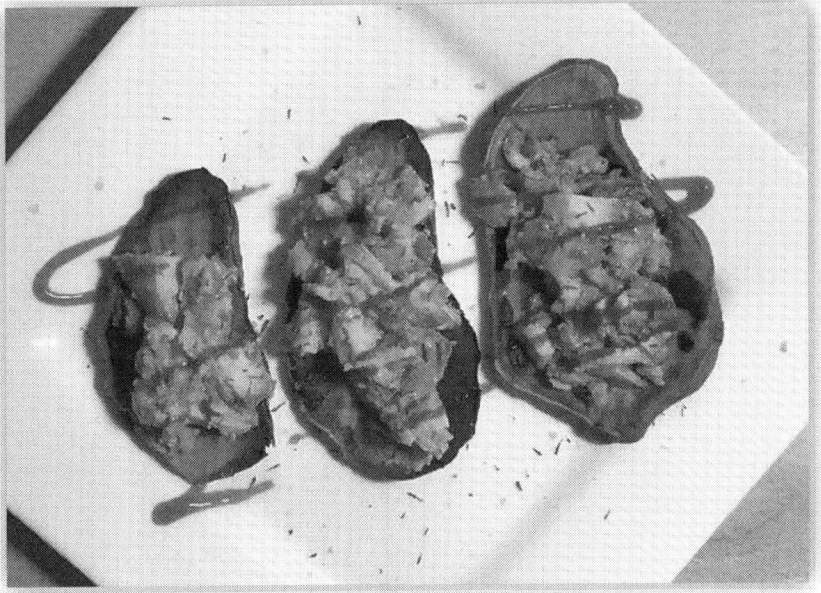

Preparation Time: 10 Minutes
Cooking Time: 10 Minutes
Servings: 5 Slices or 2 serving

Ingredients:

- 1 Sweet Potato, large
- ½ of 1 Avocado, mashed
- ¼ tsp. Red Pepper Flakes
- ¼ tsp. Black Pepper
- Dash of Salt

Method of Preparation

- Start by dividing the sweet potato lengthwise into ¼ inch slices.
- After that, place the sweet potato in the toaster for 5 minutes on high heat or until cooked.
- Next, mash the avocado and to this, spoon in the red pepper flakes, black pepper, and salt.
- Top the roasted sweet potato with the avocado topping.
- Serve and enjoy.

Tip: You can pair the sweet potato with fried eggs instead of mashed avocado mixture.

Nutritional Information per serving: (2 slices = 1 serving)

- ✓ Calories: 73Kcal
- ✓ Carbohydrates: 10.3g
- ✓ Proteins: 1.5g
- ✓ Fat: 2.2g
- ✓ Sodium: 311mg

BLT Cukes

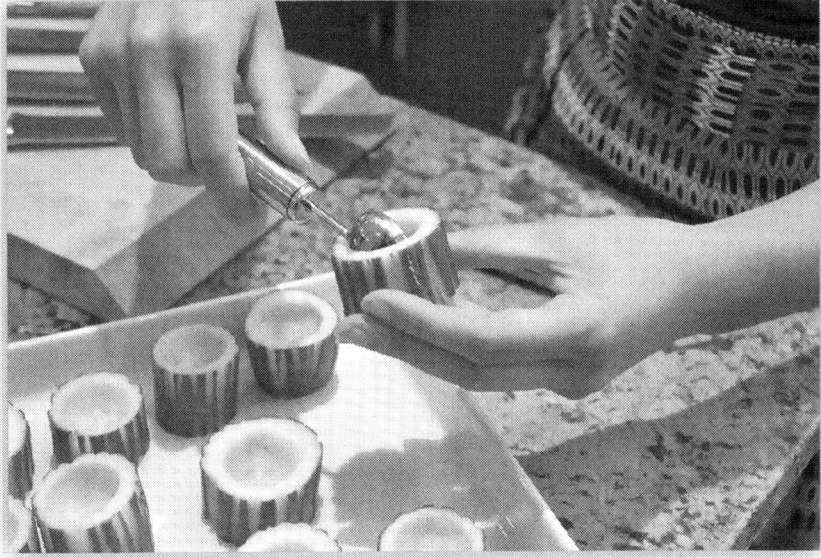

Preparation Time: 10 Minutes
Cooking Time: 10 Minutes
Servings: 8 to 10 pieces

Ingredients:

- ¼ cup Tomato, finely diced
- 1 Cucumber, large & peeled
- ½ cup Lettuce, chopped finely
- 1/8 tsp. Salt
- ½ cup Baby Spinach, finely chopped
- ¼ tsp. Salt
- 3 Bacon Slices, cooked, crisp & crumbled
- 1 tbsp. + ½ tsp. Mayonnaise

Method of Preparation

- Begin by placing lettuce, salt, spinach, pepper, bacon, mayonnaise, and tomato in a large bowl. Toss well.
- After that, trim the ends of the cucumber and slice them into two halves lengthwise.
- Next, with the help of a spoon, take out the seeds.
- Finally, spoon the bacon mixture into the cucumber pieces while mounting in the middle portion.
- Slice them into 2-inch pieces and serve.

Tip: You can top it with parsley if desired.

Nutritional Information per serving: (1 piece = 1 serving)

- ✓ Calories: 21Kcal
- ✓ Carbohydrates: 2.6g
- ✓ Proteins: 0.8g
- ✓ Fat: 1.1g
- ✓ Sodium: 62mg

Roasted Red Pepper Tapenade

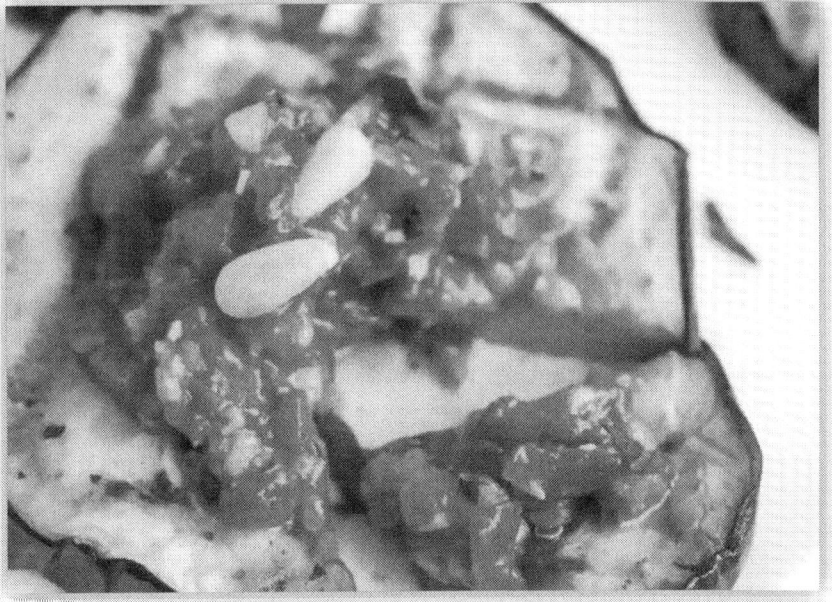

Preparation Time: 10 Minutes
Cooking Time: 10 Minutes
Servings: Makes 2 cups

Ingredients:

- 2 cups Sweet Red Peppers, toasted
- 2 tbsp. Olive Oil
- ¼ tsp. Salt
- 3 cloves of Garlic, minced
- Basil, fresh & minced
- ½ cup Almonds, blanched
- ¼ tsp. Pepper
- 1/3 cup Tomato Paste

Method of Preparation

- For making this spicy dip, place 2 cups of water in a small saucepan over medium heat.
- Boil the water, and once it starts boiling, stir in the garlic.
- Cook for 7 to 8 minutes or until tender while keeping the pan uncovered.
- Drain the water and dry the garlic with a paper towel.
- Now, blend the almonds, pepper, red pepper, salt, tomato paste, oil, and garlic in a high-speed blender for two minutes or until blended.
- After that, transfer the mixture to a medium-sized bowl and place it in the refrigerator for at least 4 hours.
- Before serving, top it with parsley.
- Pair it with vegetables of your choice.

Tip: Instead of almonds, you can also use walnuts or pecan.

Nutritional Information per serving:

- ✓ Calories: 58Kcal
- ✓ Carbohydrates: 3g
- ✓ Proteins: 1g
- ✓ Fat: 4g
- ✓ Sodium: 152mg

Kale Chips

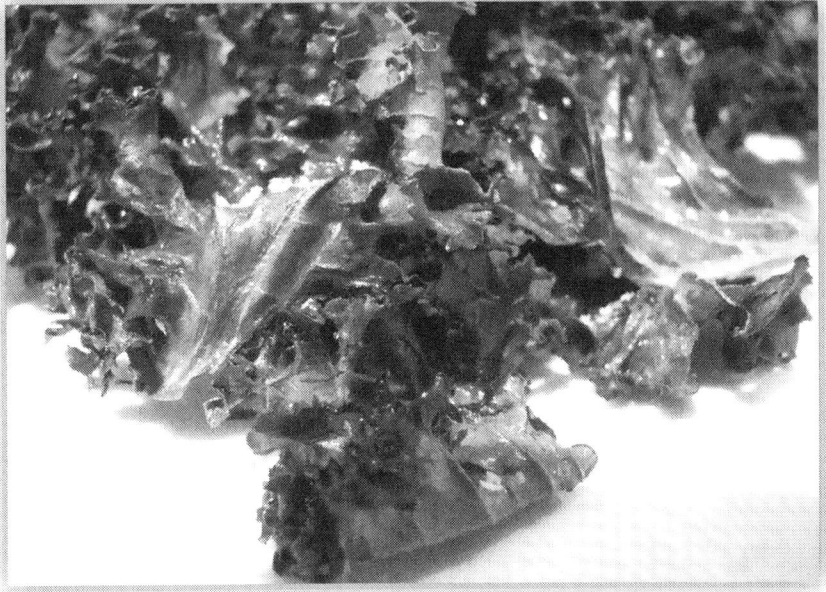

Preparation Time: 5 Minutes
Cooking Time: 25 Minutes
Servings: 4

Ingredients:

- 1 bundle of Curly Green Kale
- 1 tsp. Chili Powder
- 2 tbsp. Coconut Oil, melted

Method of Preparation

- First, preheat the oven to 225 ° F or 107 ° C.
- After that, wash the kale leaves thoroughly and pat dry the leaves. Tore them into smaller pieces. Discard the stems.
- Next, place them in a large bowl along with oil and chili powder. Toss them well. Tip: With your hands, you can massage the oil and the seasoning to the kale leaves.
- Now, arrange the kale leaves on a greased large baking sheet while leaving ample space in between.
- Bake them for 10 to 15 minutes. Turn the pans around and toss them lightly.
- Bake the kale leaves for further 15 minutes or until the leaves are crispy and light golden brown.
- Allow the baked leaves to cool slightly.
- Enjoy and serve immediately.

Tip: Instead of curly kale, you can also use purple kale.

Nutritional Information per serving:

- ✓ Calories: 50Kcal
- ✓ Carbohydrates: 3.5g
- ✓ Proteins: 1.7g
- ✓ Fat: 3.7g
- ✓ Sodium: 15mg

Autumn Fruits Salad

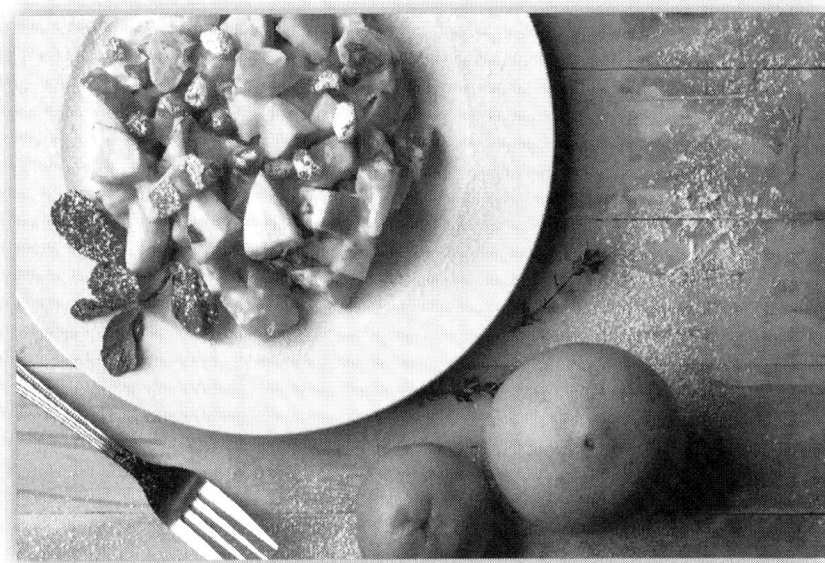

Preparation Time: 5 Minutes
Cooking Time: 10 Minutes
Servings: 4

Ingredients:

- 1 tbsp. Honey
- 1/3 cup Pecans, chopped & toasted
- 2 Pears, ripe & cubed
- ¼ cup Greek Yoghurt, plain & low-fat
- 2 tbsp. Lemon Juice

Method of Preparation

- To start with, place pears and lemon juice in a medium-sized bowl and toss them well.
- After that, stir in the pecans. Toss again.
- Now, divide the mixture among the four serving bowls.
- Next, mix yogurt and honey in another bowl until combined.
- Finally, spoon the yogurt mixture over the fruits.
- Serve cold or immediately.

Tip: If you prefer, you can even sprinkle ground cinnamon over the yogurt.

Nutritional Information per serving: (1 serving = ¾ cup salad and 1 tbsp. yogurt mixture)

- ✓ Calories: 140Kcal
- ✓ Carbohydrates: 20g
- ✓ Proteins: 3g
- ✓ Fat: 7g
- ✓ Sodium: 7mg

Roasted Radishes

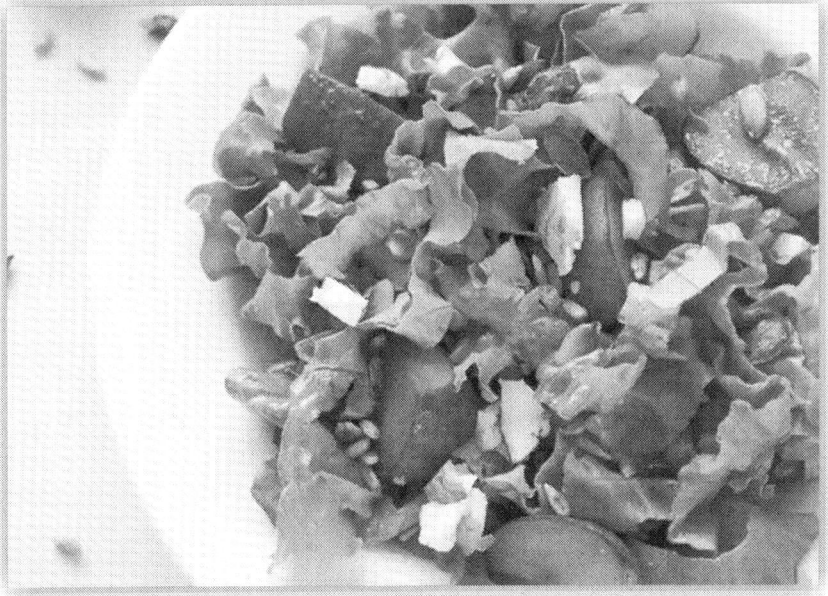

Preparation Time: 5 Minutes
Cooking Time: 25 Minutes
Servings: 4

Ingredients:

- 1 tsp. Dill Weed
- 2 tbsp. Avocado Oil
- 1 tsp. Salt
- 1 lb. Red Radishes, quartered
- ½ tsp. Parsley, dried
- ¼ tsp. Onion Powder
- ½ tsp. Garlic Powder
- ½ tsp. Black Pepper

Method of Preparation

- First, preheat the oven to 425 ° F or 218 ° C.
- Next, combine dill, onion powder, salt, pepper powder, parsley, and garlic powder in a small bowl until mixed well.
- Keep radishes along with avocado oil in a large bowl. Toss well so that the oil coats the radishes.
- Now, spoon the seasoning over the radishes and toss again.
- Then, place the seasoned radishes on a large baking sheet while leaving ample space between each of them.
- Finally, bake them for 17 to 20 minutes or until radishes are tender.

Tip: If desired, you can Italian seasoning to it.

Nutritional Information per serving:

- ✓ Calories: 52Kcal
- ✓ Carbohydrates: 4.45g
- ✓ Proteins: 0.89g
- ✓ Fat: 7g
- ✓ Sodium: 71mg

Almond Macaroons

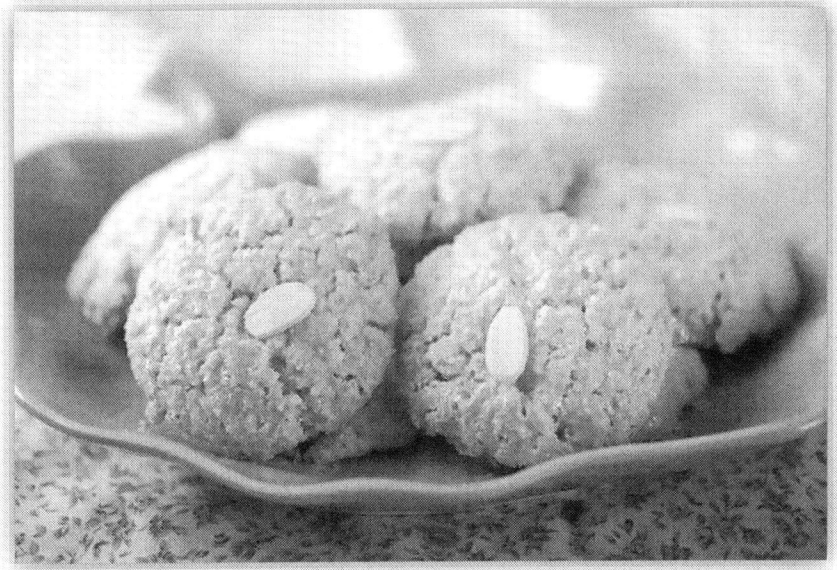

Preparation Time: 10 Minutes
Cooking Time: 1 Hour
Servings: Makes 45

Ingredients:

- 1 tbsp. Sugar-free sweetener of your choice
- 2 cups + 2 tbsp. Almond Flour
- ½ tsp. Almond Extract
- 2 Egg Whites
- ¼ cup Granulated Sweetener, sugar-free

Method of Preparation

- For making these delightful macaroons, mix the almond flour with almond extract, egg whites and sweetener until you get a dough.
- Knead the dough until it becomes smooth.
- After that, make balls out of this dough, which is about 1-inch.
- Next, arrange the balls on the parchment paper-lined baking sheet and bake them for 55 to 60 minutes.
- Take the baking sheet from the oven and allow it to cool completely.
- Finally, sprinkle the granulated sweetener over the top of the macaroons.

Tip: If preferred, you can add chopped nuts to it.

Nutritional Information per serving:

- ✓ Calories: 29Kcal
- ✓ Carbohydrates: 2g
- ✓ Proteins: 1g
- ✓ Fat: 3g
- ✓ Sodium: 1mg

Pumpkin Muffins

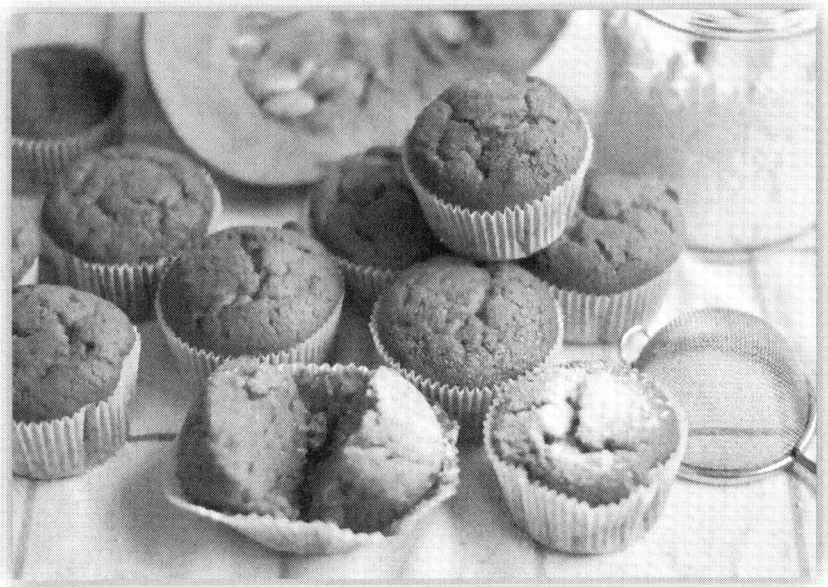

Preparation Time: 10 Minutes
Cooking Time: 25 Minutes
Servings: Makes 10

Ingredients:

- 1 tsp. Vanilla Extract
- ½ cup Coconut Flour
- ½ cup Butter or Ghee
- ½ cup Almond Flour, blanched
- ¾ cup Pumpkin Puree
- 2/3 cup Erythritol
- 4 Eggs, large
- 1 tbsp. Pumpkin Spice
- 1 tbsp. Baking Powder, gluten-free
- ¼ tsp. Salt

Method of Preparation

- Preheat the oven to 350 ° F or 150 ° C.
- Next, mix all the dry ingredients in a large bowl until well incorporated.
- After that, whisk all the wet ingredients in another bowl until mixed well.
- Now, stir in the dry ingredients to the wet ingredients.
- Give a good stir until everything comes together.
- Now, spoon the batter into the muffins cups evenly about ¾th full.
- Finally, bake them for 20 to 25 minutes or until a toothpick inserted in the center comes clean and is golden colored.

Tip: If you prefer, you can add pumpkin seeds to it.

Nutritional Information per serving: (1 serving = 1 muffin)

- ✓ Calories: 173Kcal
- ✓ Carbohydrates: 4g
- ✓ Proteins: 4g
- ✓ Fat: 14g
- ✓ Sodium: 23mg

Sautéed Shrimp

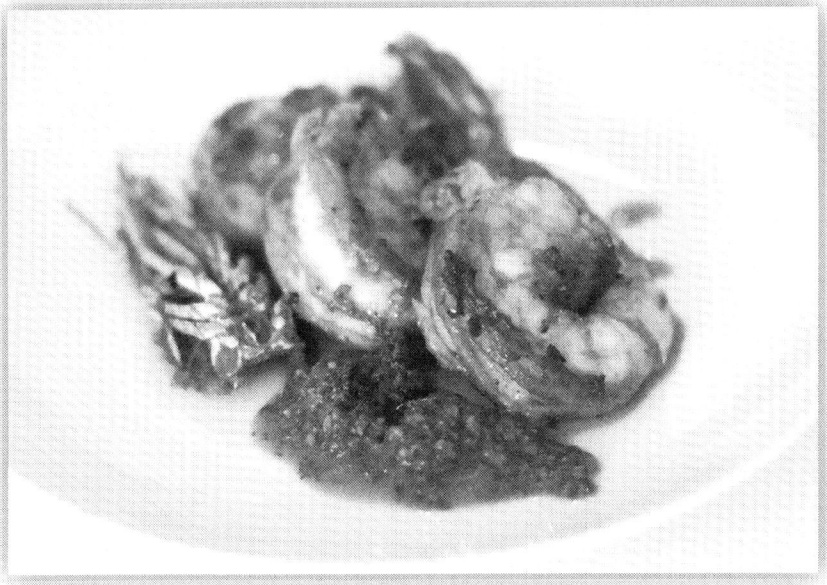

Preparation Time: 10 Minutes
Cooking Time: 45 Minutes
Servings: Makes 18

Ingredients:

- 2/3 cup Cider Vinegar
- 12 cups Water
- 1 cup Green Bell Pepper, chopped
- ¼ tsp. Black Pepper
- 2 lb. Shrimp, unpeeled & shrimp
- 1 ½ tbsp. Vegetable Oil
- 2 tsp. Old Bay Seasoning
- ½ tsp. Salt
- 1 cup Onion, chopped

Method of Preparation

- Start by heating water in a large saucepan over medium-high heat.
- Once it starts boiling, stir in the shrimp and cook them for 3 minutes or until cooked. Drain the water and cool it.
- Next, keep the shrimp in a large zip lock bag.
- To this, spoon in all the remaining ingredients and seal the bag. Shake them well.
- Marinate them for half an hour in the refrigerator while tossing the bag occasionally.
- Once the time is up, remove the shrimp from the marinade.
- Peel the shrimp and keep it in a bowl.
- Finally, stir in the marinade and remix them.

Tip: Make sure to not mix the marinade with the shrimp one to two hours before it is to be served.

Nutritional Information per serving:

- ✓ Calories: 57Kcal
- ✓ Carbohydrates: 2.1g
- ✓ Proteins: 7.9g
- ✓ Fat: 1.8g
- ✓ Sodium: 260mg

Grilled Peaches

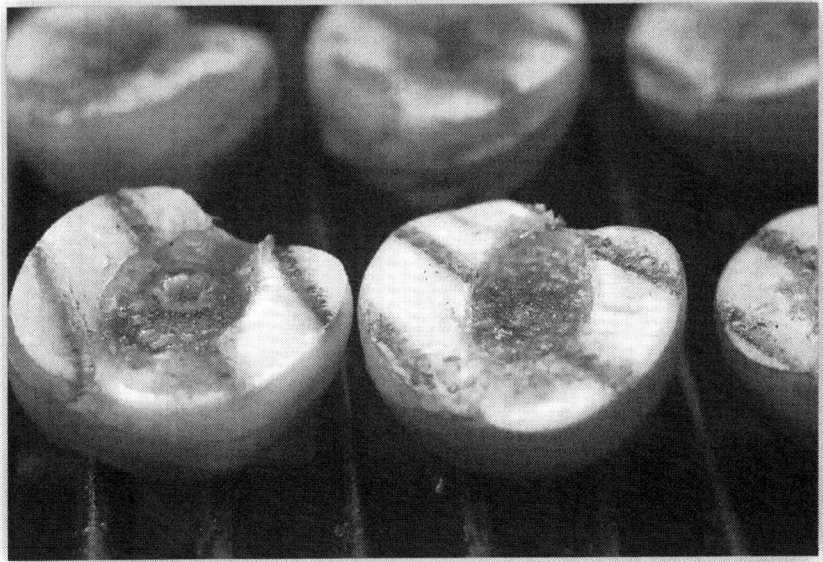

Preparation Time: 5 Minutes
Cooking Time: 8 Minutes
Servings: 4

Ingredients:

- 2 Peaches, large
- 2 tbsp. Extra Virgin Olive Oil

Method of Preparation

- To start with, preheat the gas grill to medium heat.
- After that, slice the peaches into two halves along the seam.
- Now, brush the peaches with ½ tbsp. of olive oil along the halves.
- Next, place the peaches on the grill with the cut side down.
- Cook for 4 minutes and turn them over.
- Cook them again for another 4 minutes.
- Remove them from the grill and peel off the skin.

Tip: You can also use nectarines.

Nutritional Information per serving:

- ✓ Calories: 94Kcal
- ✓ Carbohydrates: 8g
- ✓ Proteins: 1g
- ✓ Fat: 7g
- ✓ Sodium: 166mg

Eggplant Chips

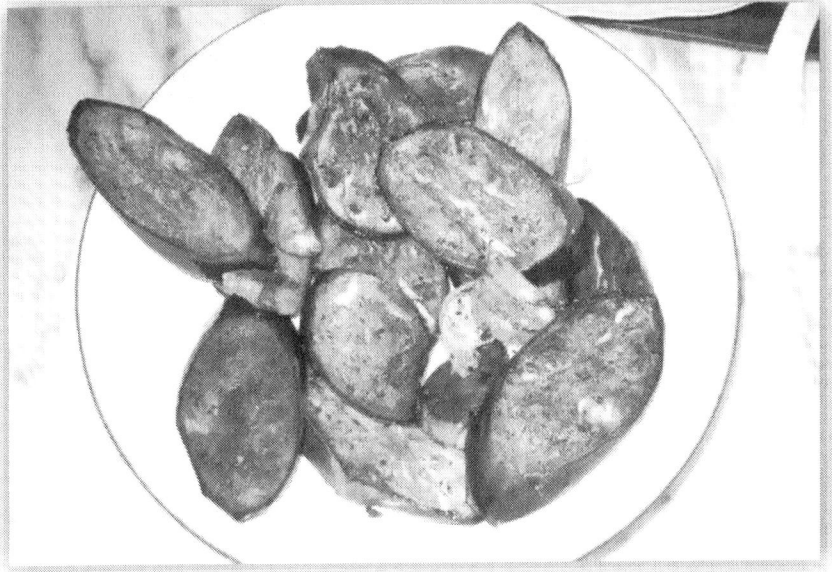

Preparation Time: 5 Minutes
Cooking Time: 8 Minutes
Servings: 8

Ingredients:

- 2 Japanese Eggplants
- 1 tbsp. Garam Masala
- 1 tbsp. Salt
- 3 tbsp. Olive Oil

Method of Preparation

- Preheat the oven to 350 ° F or 175 °C.
- After that, slice the eggplants, which are ¼ inch.
- Now, arrange the eggplant slices in a large baking sheet in a single layer.
- Next, sprinkle the salt and black pepper over it and allow it to sit for an hour.
- Pat dry the slices with a paper towel.
- Then, mix garam masala and olive oil in another bowl until combined.
- Brush the spice mixture over the eggplant slices and return the slices to the sheet.
- Finally, bake them for 25 to 30 minutes or until they are crisp and browned.
- Remove them from the oven. Serve warm.

Tip: You can serve along with curd.

Nutritional Information per serving:

- ✓ Calories: 94Kcal
- ✓ Carbohydrates: 8g
- ✓ Proteins: 1g
- ✓ Fat: 7g
- ✓ Sodium: 166mg

Fennel Kale Slaw

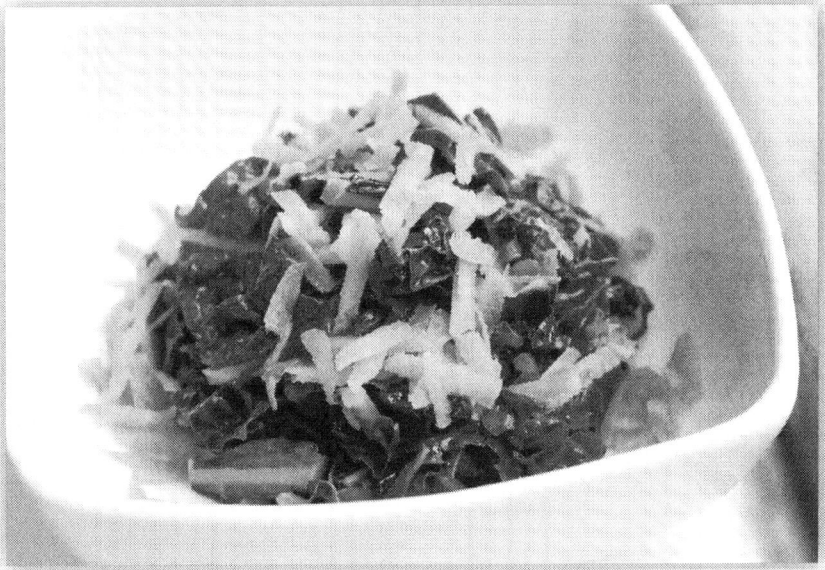

Preparation Time: 5 Minutes
Cooking Time: 15 Minutes
Servings: 2

Ingredients:

- 2 Carrots, small & shredded
- ½ tbsp. Extra Virgin Olive Oil
- ¼ Fennel Bulb - sliced thinly
- ½ tbsp. Lemon Juice
- 2 Kale Stalks - leaves chopped
- Black Pepper, freshly ground, as needed
- 1/8 tsp. Salt

Method of Preparation

- To start with, combine the carrots with the kale and fennel.
- After that, whisk olive, salt, lime juice, and pepper in another small bowl.
- Now, drizzle the olive oil mixture over the carrot kale mixture.
- Toss well and serve immediately.

Tip: Instead of lemon juice, you can also use key lime.

Nutritional Information per serving:

- ✓ Calories: 72Kcal
- ✓ Carbohydrates: 9g
- ✓ Proteins: 2g
- ✓ Fat: 3.7g
- ✓ Sodium: 199mg

Cauliflower Rice Salad

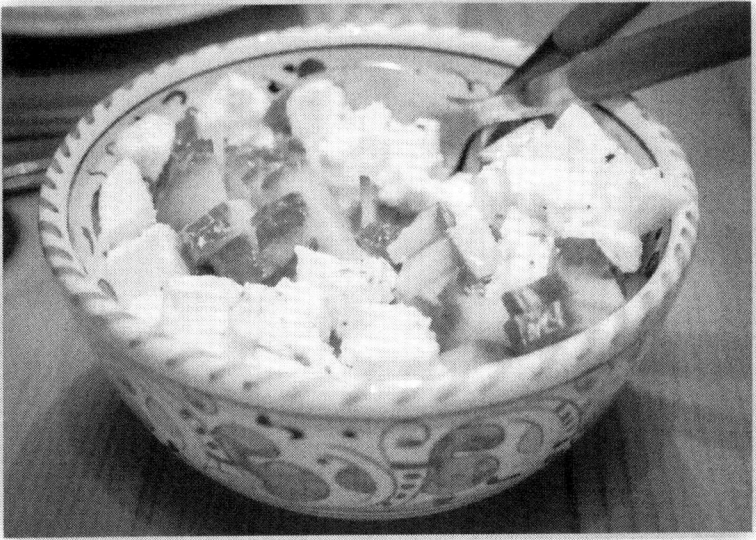

Preparation Time: 15 Minutes
Cooking Time: 30 Minutes
Servings: 4

Ingredients:

- 1 Cauliflower, medium & torn into florets
- ¼ cup Carrot, shredded
- 1 cup Lettuce, shredded
- ½ cup Green Beans, fresh & sliced into 1-inch
- ¼ tsp. Black Pepper
- ½ cup Mayonnaise, fat-free
- ¼ tsp. Salt
- 2 Tomatoes, medium & diced
- 1 Garlic clove, minced
- ¼ cup Red Onion, chopped finely
- 2 tbsp. Cilantro, chopped
- ¼ tsp. Red Chili Powder

Method of Preparation

- To begin with, heat water in a deep saucepan over medium-high heat.
- Next, stir in the cauliflower and green beans to it.
- Cook them for 5 to 8 minutes or until cooked. Drain the water.
- Meanwhile, mix all the remaining ingredients, excluding the lettuce in another bowl until combined well.
- Finally, spoon the cauliflower and green beans to this mixture along with lettuce.
- Place it in the refrigerator for 1 hour before serving.

Tip: Instead of mayonnaise, you can also use plain yogurt.

Nutritional Information per serving:

- ✓ Calories: 30Kcal
- ✓ Carbohydrates: 6g
- ✓ Proteins: 1g
- ✓ Fat: 0g
- ✓ Sodium: 135mg

Cinnamon Coconut Lemon Balls

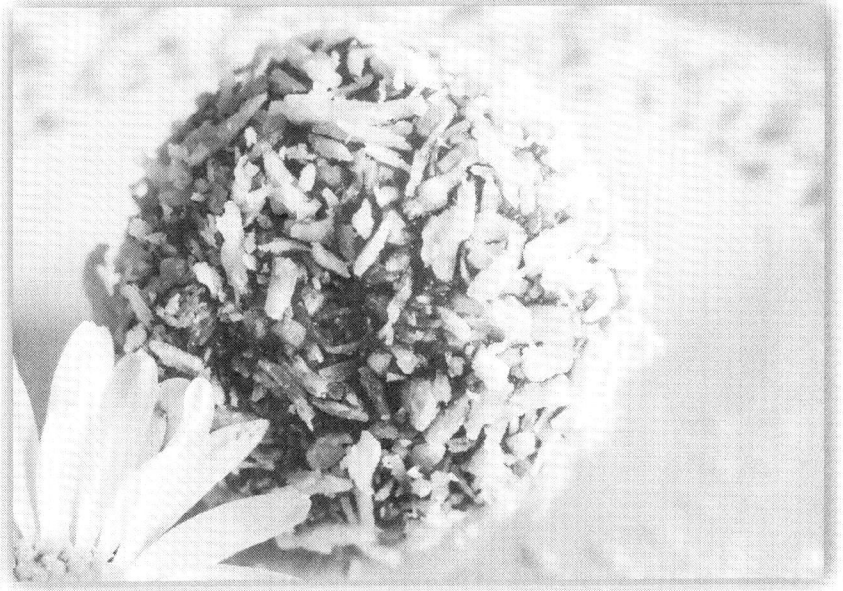

Preparation Time: 5 Minutes
Cooking Time: 8 Minutes
Servings: Makes 20 balls

Ingredients:

- 2 tbsp. Almond Oil
- ¼ cup Shredded Coconut, unsweetened
- 2 cups Almond Flour, fine
- 1 tsp. Cinnamon, grounded
- ¼ cup Maple Syrup
- 2 tsp. Lemon Zest
- ¼ tsp. Salt

Method of Preparation

- First, mix maple syrup, cinnamon, almond flour, lemon zest, and almond oil in a large mixing bowl until everything is well incorporated and you get a sticky dough.
- After that, using plastic wrap, line the large baking sheet.
- Next, divide the dough into 20 balls.
- Now, arrange the almond balls on a plate and coat it with shredded coconut.
- Serve immediately or cold.

Tip: Instead of almond oil, you can also use coconut oil.

Nutritional Information per serving:

- ✓ Calories: 97Kcal
- ✓ Carbohydrates: 6g
- ✓ Proteins: 3g
- ✓ Fat: 8g
- ✓ Sodium: 34mg

Buffalo Chicken

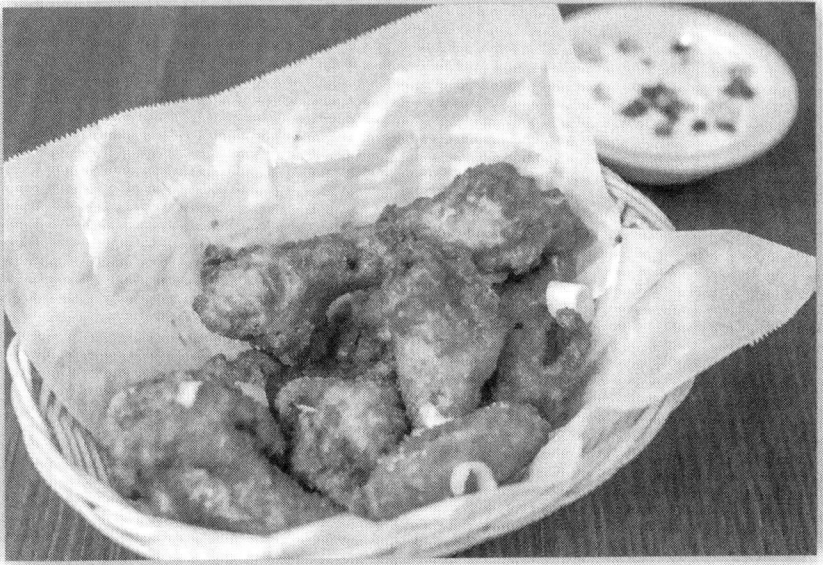

Preparation Time: 10 Minutes
Cooking Time: 40 Minutes
Servings: Makes 42

Ingredients:

- ½ cup Red Hot Sauce
- 1 lb. Chicken Breasts, cooked & sliced into chunks
- 2 tsp. Parsley, dried
- ¼ tsp. Garlic Powder
- 3 tbsp. Margarine, melted
- Cooking Spray, as needed
- Celery Sticks, as needed

Method of Preparation

- For making this highly popular recipe, you need to first preheat the oven to 350 ° F or 175 °C.
- After that, place the chicken pieces on a baking dish.
- To this, stir in the hot sauce, garlic powder, margarine, and parsley. Mix well.
- Then, pour this dressing over the chicken pieces. Toss well.
- Next, transfer the chicken pieces to the baking sheet and cook them for 18 to 20 minutes.
- Now, insert a toothpick into the middle portion of the chicken piece and see whether cooked.
- Serve it hot along with celery stalks.

Tip: You can either use ranch dressing or blue cheese dressing.

Nutritional Information per serving:

- ✓ Calories: 154Kcal
- ✓ Carbohydrates: 1g
- ✓ Proteins: 24g
- ✓ Fat: 6g
- ✓ Sodium: 209mg

Fruit & Nut Trail Mix

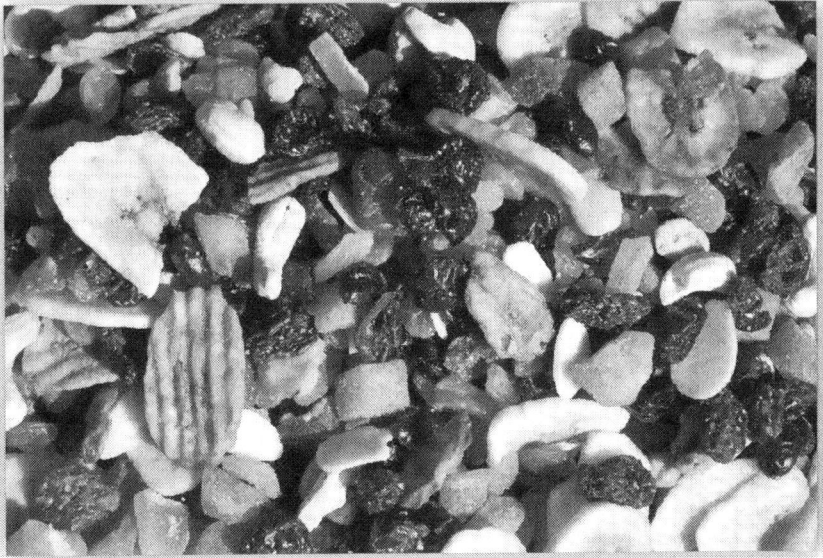

Preparation Time: 10 Minutes
Cooking Time: 10 Minutes
Servings: Makes 1 ¾ cup

Ingredients:

- ¼ cup Banana Chips
- ¼ cup Almonds, raw
- ¼ cup Apricots, dried
- ¼ cup Cashews, raw
- ¼ cup Raisins, golden
- ¼ cup Walnut, halves & raw
- Dash of Sea Salt

Method of Preparation

- Preheat the oven to 350 ° F or 175 ° C.
- After that, place the nuts and salt in a large bowl and toss them well.
- Next, transfer them to a large baking sheet and toast for 10 minutes or until it becomes golden in color while stirring them once halfway.
- Take the baking sheet from the oven and allow it to cool completely.
- Finally, combine the nuts and dried fruits.

Tip: You can either use ranch dressing or blue cheese dressing.

Nutritional Information per serving:

- ✓ Calories: 98Kcal
- ✓ Carbohydrates: 7g
- ✓ Proteins: 2.8g
- ✓ Fat: 6.7g
- ✓ Sodium: 37mg

Lemon Bread

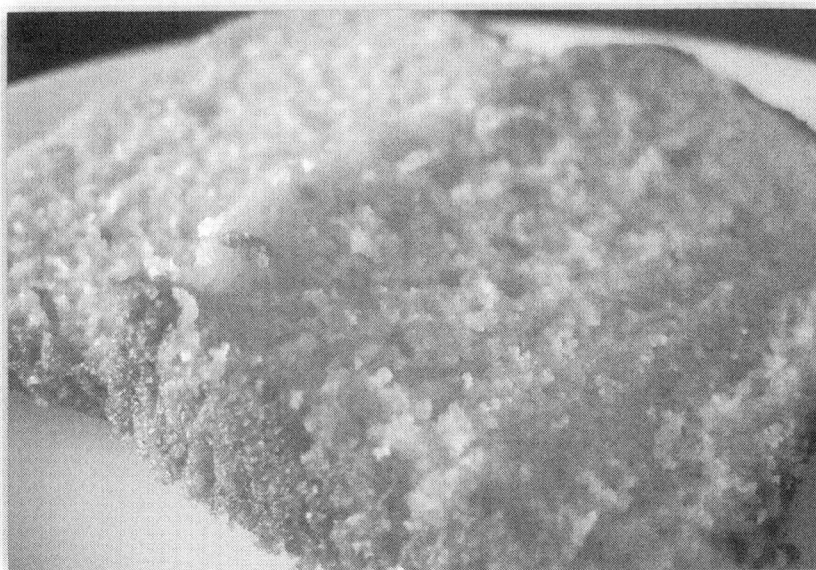

Preparation Time: 10 Minutes
Cooking Time: 40 Minutes
Servings: 10

Ingredients:

- 4 ½ tbsp. Lemon Juice, fresh
- 1 cup Granulated Low Carb Sweetener
- 1/3 cup Granulated Low Carb Sweetener for the glaze
- 1 ½ tsp. Lemon Peel, grated
- ½ cup Egg Whites, large & beaten lightly
- ½ cup Skim Milk
- 1 ½ cup Low Carb Flour
- ½ tsp. Salt
- 1 tsp. Baking Powder
- ½ cup Margarine, melted

Method of Preparation

- Preheat the oven to 350 ° F or 175 ° C.
- After that, combine the sweetener, butter, and egg whites in another bowl until mixed well.
- To this, stir in all the remaining ingredients and give a good stir until everything comes together.
- Now, transfer the mixture to a greased parchment paper-lined baking pan.
- Then, bake for 44 to 50 minutes or until a skewer inserted in the middle portion comes clean.
- Next, poke holes randomly across the cake.
- Once poked, to make the drizzle, mix the sweetener and lime juice in a small saucepan.
- Cook for 3 minutes over medium heat or until the sweetener is dissolved.
- When slightly cooled, spoon the drizzle over the cake slowly.
- Cool the bread in the pan for another 20 minutes.

Tip: You can you butterlike also instead of margarine.

Nutritional Information per serving:

- ✓ Calories: 157Kcal
- ✓ Carbohydrates: 15g
- ✓ Proteins: 4g
- ✓ Fat: 1g
- ✓ Sodium: 230mg

Tropical Tofu Shake

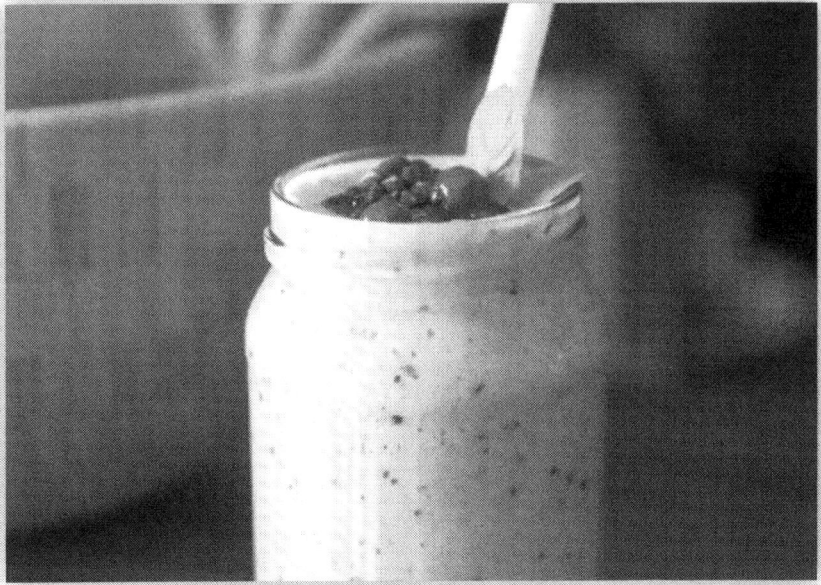

Preparation Time: 10 Minutes
Cooking Time: 10 Minutes
Servings: 3

Ingredients:

- 2 tsp. Honey
- 16 oz. Tofu, silken & drained
- 1 Banana
- 1 ½ cup Coconut Water
- 1 cup Strawberries, frozen & whole

Method of Preparation

- For making this delicious smoothie, all you need to do is to blend all the ingredients in a high-speed blender.
- Blend for two minutes or until you get a smooth mixture.
- Transfer to a serving glass.
- Enjoy it cold or immediately.

Tip: You can use your favorite fruit instead of banana.

Nutritional Information per serving:

✓ Calories: 148Kcal
✓ Carbohydrates: 26g
✓ Proteins: 10g
✓ Fat: 2g
✓ Sodium: 131mg

Egg Muffins

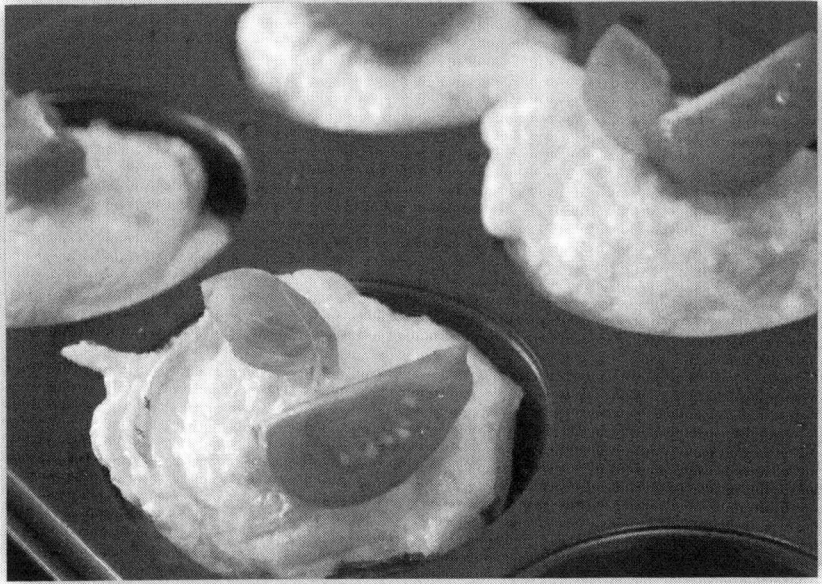

Preparation Time: 7 Minutes
Cooking Time: 25 Minutes
Servings: 4

Ingredients:

- ½ of 1 Onion, diced
- 1/8 tsp. Sea Salt
- 8 Cherry Tomatoes
- 1 tsp. Olive Oil
- 3 tbsp. Milk
- 1 ½ cups Kale, chopped
- 5 Eggs, preferably farm-raised
- Black Pepper, freshly grounded

Method of Preparation

- Preheat the oven to 350 ° F or 175 ° C.
- After that, whisk the eggs with milk, salt, and pepper in a medium-sized bowl until mixed well.
- Now, spoon the olive oil into a large saucepan and heat it over medium-high heat.
- Once the oil becomes hot, stir in the onions and sauté them for 3 to 4 minutes or until softened.
- To this, add the kale and cook for 1 minute or until wilted.
- Then, add the onion and kale into the egg mixture and beat the mixture well until everything is well incorporated.
- Now, lightly grease the muffin pans with oil.
- Pour the mixture to the greased muffin pans evenly.
- Top each of the muffin mixtures with four halved cherry tomatoes.
- Finally, bake them for 23 to 25 minutes or until browned on top and puffy.
- Allow them to cool slightly before serving.

Tip: You can add other veggies like mushroom also to the mixture.

Nutritional Information per serving:

- ✓ Calories: 112Kcal
- ✓ Carbohydrates: 5g
- ✓ Proteins: 9g
- ✓ Fat: 7g
- ✓ Sodium: 93mg

Carrot Apple Juice

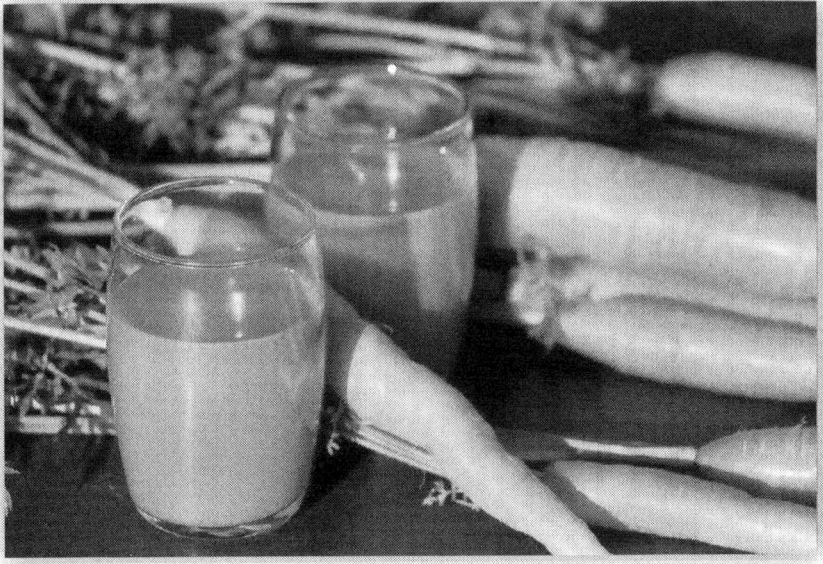

Preparation Time: 5 Minutes
Cooking Time: 3 Minutes
Servings: 2

Ingredients:

- 1 Carrot, medium & sliced into halves
- 1 cup Ice Cubes
- ½ cup Cold Water
- 1 Apple, small & seeded
- 1 Orange, halved & seeded
- ½ inch thick Pineapple slice, peeled

Method of Preparation

- To begin with, combine all the ingredients needed to make the juice in a high-speed blender.
- Blend them for a minute or two or until smooth.
- Serve immediately.

Tip: You can add sweetener if needed.

Nutritional Information per serving:

✓ Calories: 85Kcal
✓ Carbohydrates: 22g
✓ Proteins: 1g
✓ Fat: 0g
✓ Sodium: 22mg

Spinach Dip with Greek Yoghurt

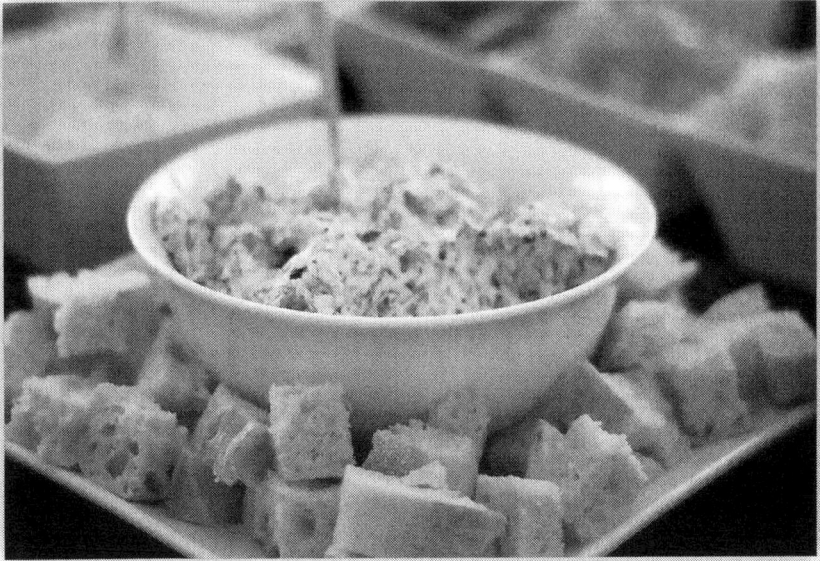

Preparation Time: 5 Minutes
Cooking Time: 5 Minutes
Servings: 2 cups

Ingredients:

- 3 tbsp. Mint, chopped
- 1 cup Spinach, frozen
- ½ cup Parsley, chopped
- 2 cloves of Garlic
- 1 tbsp. Zaatar
- 1 tsp. Salt
- 2 tbsp. Lemon Juice
- 2 cups Greek Yoghurt, fat-free

Method of Preparation

- First, place the spinach in the microwave and defrost it.
- After that, keep the garlic cloves and salt in a mortar and pestle. Crush it.
- Next, combine za'atar, yogurt, and lime juice in another bowl, and to this, spoon in the garlic paste. Mix well.
- Then, add the herbs while reserving a tablespoon.
- Place in a cool place for two hours or more.

Tip: Pair it with vegetable sticks.

Nutritional Information per serving:

- ✓ Calories: 174Kcal
- ✓ Carbohydrates: 18g
- ✓ Proteins: 27g
- ✓ Fat: 1g
- ✓ Sodium: 53mg

Applesauce Pancakes

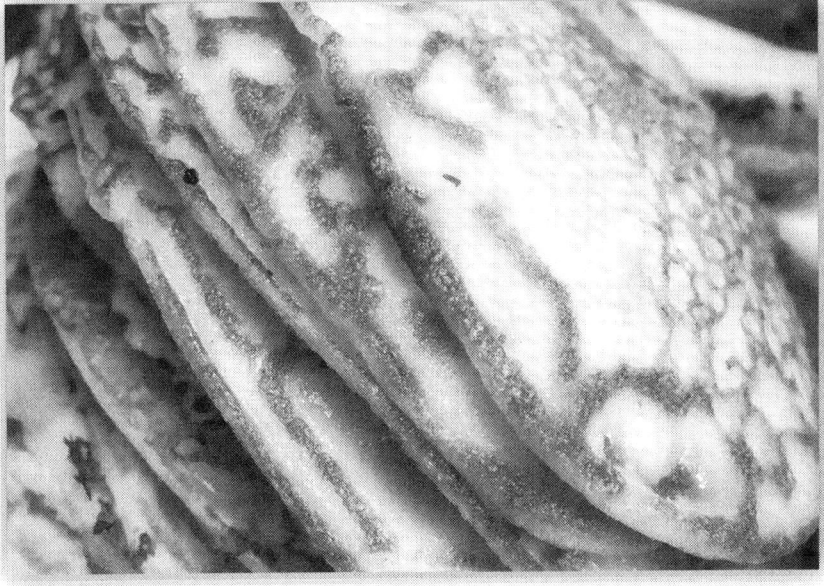

Preparation Time: 10 Minutes
Cooking Time: 5 Minutes
Servings: Makes 10

Ingredients:

- ¼ cup Applesauce, unsweetened
- 1 cup Gluten-free Flour
- 1 cup Buttermilk, non-fat
- 1 Egg, large & beaten lightly
- 2 tbsp. Wheat Germ, toasted
- 1 tsp. Baking Soda
- 2 tsp. Vegetable Oil
- 1/8 tsp. Salt

Method of Preparation

- For making these flavourful pancakes, mix flour, salt, wheat germ, and baking soda in a large bowl until combined well.
- After that, make a well in the middle portion of the bowl.
- Next, stir together buttermilk, applesauce, egg, and vegetable oil in another bowl.
- Then, add the flour mixture to the buttermilk mixture.
- Give a good stir so that everything comes together.
- Now, heat a non-stick pan over medium heat.
- Brush it with oil and then scoop ¼ cup of batter into the hot skillet while spreading it out into a circle.
- Cook them for 4 minutes. bubbles will form while the edges are getting browned.
- Flip the pancakes. Cook for one minute.
- Serve and enjoy.

Tip: You can serve it along with fruits.

Nutritional Information per serving:

- ✓ Calories: 74Kcal
- ✓ Carbohydrates: 11.5g
- ✓ Proteins: 3g
- ✓ Fat: 1.8g
- ✓ Sodium: 143mg

Sesame Breadsticks

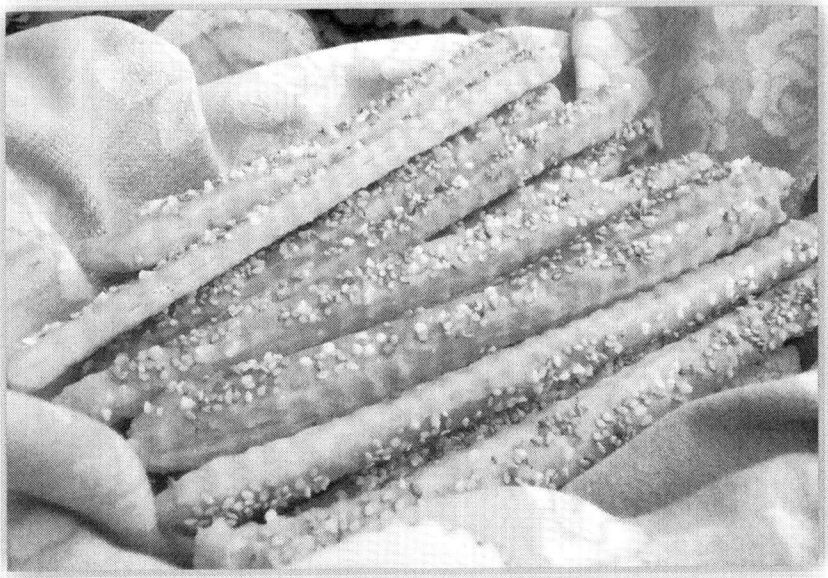

Preparation Time: 10 Minutes
Cooking Time: 5 Minutes
Servings: Makes 10

Ingredients:

- 1 tsp. Thyme, dried
- ½ cup Almond Meal
- 1 tbsp. Olive Oil
- ½ cup Arrowroot Flour
- ¼ cup Almond Milk
- ¼ tsp. Baking Soda
- ½ tsp. Garlic, granulated
- ¼ tsp. Salt
- 2 tbsp. Sesame Seeds

Method of Preparation

- Preheat the oven to 350 ° F or 175 ° C.
- Next, combine all the ingredients needed to make the breadsticks in a large bowl until it becomes a smooth dough.
- After that, make ten balls out of this dough and then roll each of them into 4-inch sticks.
- Now, arrange the sticks on the greased parchment paper-lined baking sheet.
- Then, brush the sticks with the olive oil and sprinkle some extra sesame seeds.
- Finally, bake them for 13 to 15 minutes or until they are golden in color.
- Allow them to cool completely before serving.

Tip: You can serve it along with fruits.

Nutritional Information per serving:

✓ Calories: 69Kcal
✓ Carbohydrates: 5.9g
✓ Proteins: 1.9g
✓ Fat: 4.3g
✓ Sodium: 45.2mg

Granola Bars

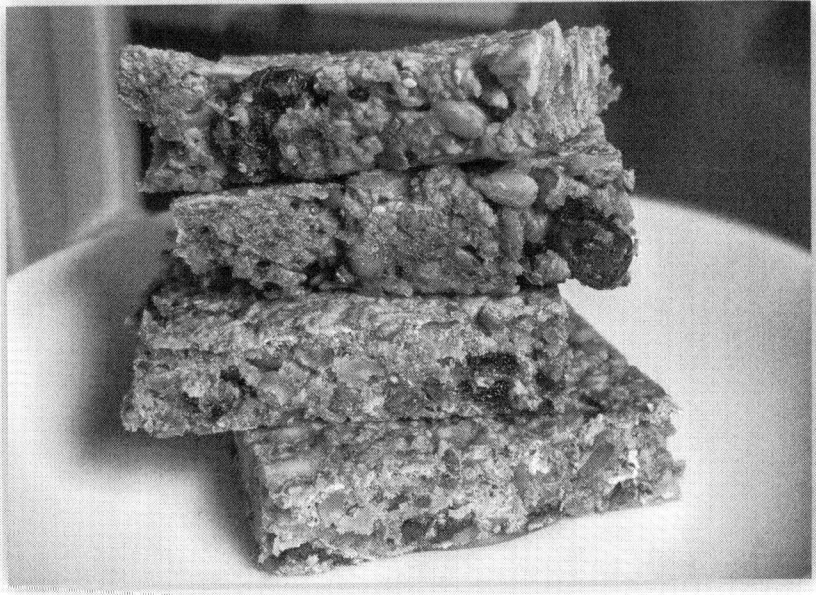

Preparation Time: 15 Minutes
Cooking Time: 20 Minutes
Servings: Makes 12 Bars

Ingredients:

- 2 cups Granola, low-fat
- 1 Egg, large + 1 Egg White, beaten lightly
- 2 tbsp. Stevia
- 1 tsp. Almond Extract
- ¼ cup Cranberries, unsweetened & dried
- ½ tsp. Cinnamon, grounded
- ¼ cup Almonds, chopped

Method of Preparation

- Preheat the oven to 350 ° F or 175 ° C.
- After that, mix granola, cranberries, cinnamon, stevia, and cinnamon in a bowl until combined well.
- Next, spoon the almond extract to the lightly beaten egg.
- Then, stir the egg mixture to the granola mixture and give everything a good stir.
- Now, pour the mixture to a greased baking sheet and spread it evenly.
- Bake the mixture for 23 minutes or until browned lightly.
- Allow it to cool completely before serving.
- With the aid of a parchment paper, lift the bars from the oven.
- Slice the bars and enjoy them.

Tip: You can store in an air-tight container for 2 to 3 weeks.

Nutritional Information per serving:

- ✓ Calories: 80Kcal
- ✓ Carbohydrates: 12g
- ✓ Proteins: 3g
- ✓ Fat: 2.5g
- ✓ Sodium: 40mg

Bacon-Wrapped Dates

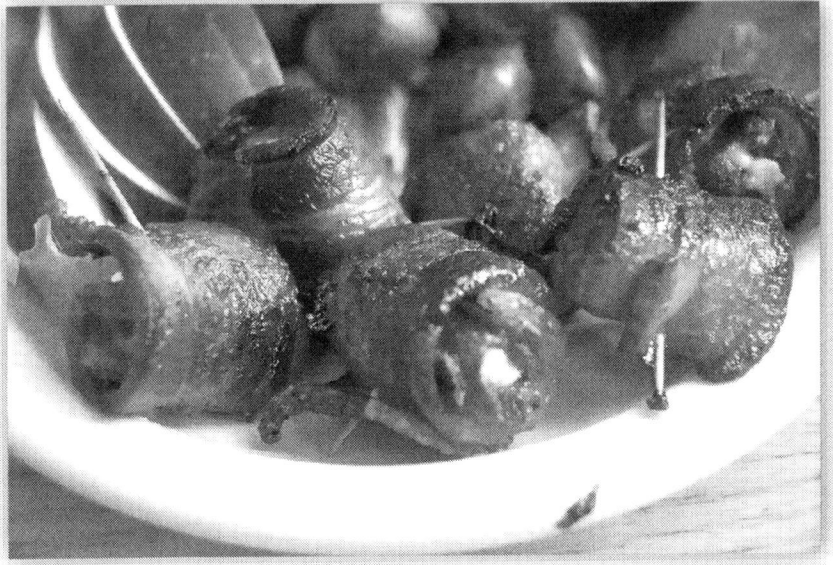

Preparation Time: 10 Minutes
Cooking Time: 10 Minutes
Servings: 24

Ingredients:

- 24 Dates, whole & pitted
- 12 Bacon Slices, sliced into halves

For the filling:

- 24 Almonds, whole

Method of Preparation

- To start with, preheat the oven to 400 ° F or 200 ° C.
- After that, soak the toothpicks in a bowl of water.
- Next, slit open the date and fill them with one almond.
- Then, slice the bacon into two halves and wrap one half of the bacon over the date.
- Secure it with a toothpick and place them on a baking tray with the seal side down.
- Finally, bake them for 12 to 15 minutes or until they are crisp.

Tip: Instead of almond, you can use goat cheese also.

Nutritional Information per serving:

- ✓ Calories: 71Kcal
- ✓ Carbohydrates: 5g
- ✓ Proteins: 1g
- ✓ Fat: 4g
- ✓ Sodium: 72mg

Gazpacho

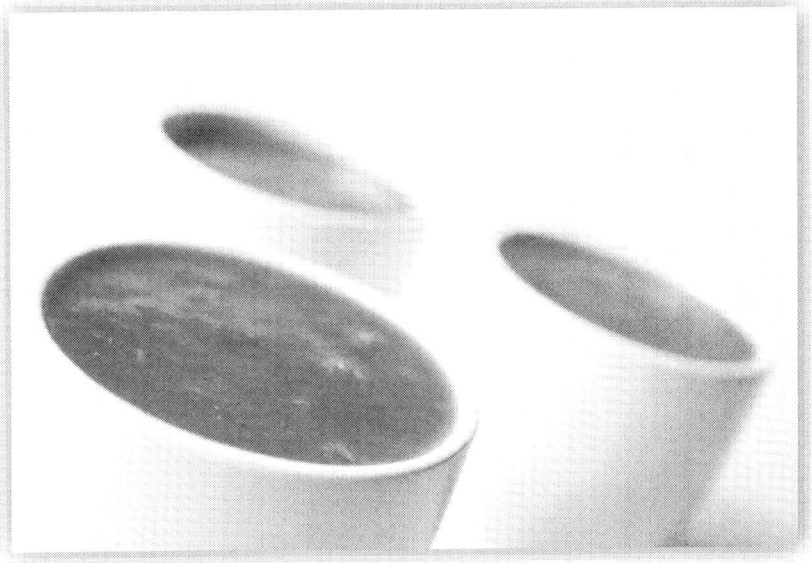

Preparation Time: 10 Minutes
Cooking Time: 10 Minutes
Servings: 6

Ingredients:

- 1 cup Yellow Bell Pepper, chopped
- 3 ½ cups Yellow Tomato, chopped & seeded
- 2 tbsp. White Wine Vinegar
- 2 cups Cucumber, chopped, seeded & peeled
- 1 tbsp. Honey
- ½ cup Red Bell Pepper, chopped
- 1 tbsp. Mint, fresh & chopped
- ½ cup Red Onion, chopped
- ¼ tsp. Cumin, grounded
- 2 tsp. Extra Virgin Olive Oil
- 1 tbsp. Cilantro, fresh & chopped

Method of Preparation

- To start with, place yellow tomato, red bell pepper, cucumber, green bell pepper, yellow bell pepper, red onion, and garlic in a high-speed blender.
- Blend them for a minute or two or until you get a smooth mixture.
- Next, stir in mint and all the remaining ingredients to the blender.
- Pulse them for 5 minutes or until mixed well.
- Finally, transfer the mixture to a bowl and cover it well.
- Place the soup in the refrigerator for at least an hour and serve.

Tip: If you would like it spicier, you can add jalapeno.

Nutritional Information per serving:

- ✓ Calories: 77Kcal
- ✓ Carbohydrates: 13.9g
- ✓ Proteins: 2.9g
- ✓ Fat: 2.3g
- ✓ Sodium: 342mg

Stuffed Mushrooms

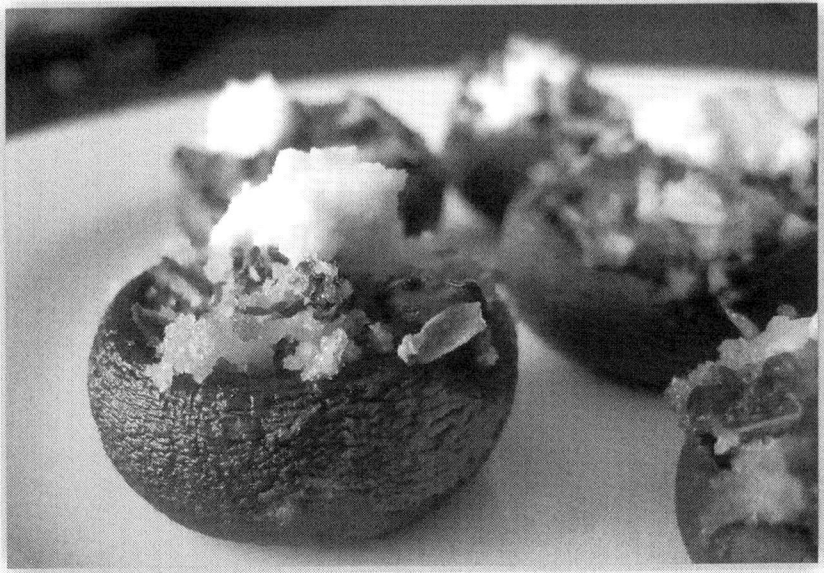

Preparation Time: 10 Minutes
Cooking Time: 60 Minutes
Servings: 6

Ingredients:

- 1 tbsp. Parmesan Cheese, grated
- 6 Mushrooms, extra-large & white
- 1 tbsp. Mozzarella Cheese, grated & reduced-fat
- 2 tsp. Balsamic Vinegar
- 2 tbsp. Bread Crumbs
- 2 tsp. Olive Oil, divided
- 2 oz. Turkey Sausage Patties - crumbled
- ¼ of 1 Onion, small & diced
- ¼ of 1 Green Bell Pepper, small & diced

Method of Preparation

- First, preheat the oven to 325 ° F or 190 ° C.
- After that, cut the stems of the mushrooms and chop them up. Keep it aside.
- Next, keep the mushroom heads in a large bowl along with vinegar and olive oil. Toss well. Set it aside.
- Then, heat one tsp. of olive oil in a medium-sized skillet over medium-high heat.
- To this, stir in the onion, mushrooms stems, and green pepper.
- Cook them for 3 minutes and stir in the sausage.
- Sauté them for 9 to 10 minutes or until the mushrooms are browned while stirring occasionally.
- Now, spoon in the bread crumbs and give everything a good stir.
- Finally, spoon in the mozzarella cheese into it and mix well until the cheese is melted.
- Off the heat and add parmesan cheese to the mixture.
- Spoon the sausage mixture to each of the mushroom caps and arrange them on a baking dish.
- Bake for 42 minutes or until the top portion becomes crispy.

Tip: If you would like it spicier, you can add jalapeno.

Nutritional Information per serving:

- ✓ Calories: 60Kcal
- ✓ Carbohydrates: 4g
- ✓ Proteins: 4g
- ✓ Fat: 3g
- ✓ Sodium: 100mg

Zucchini Chips

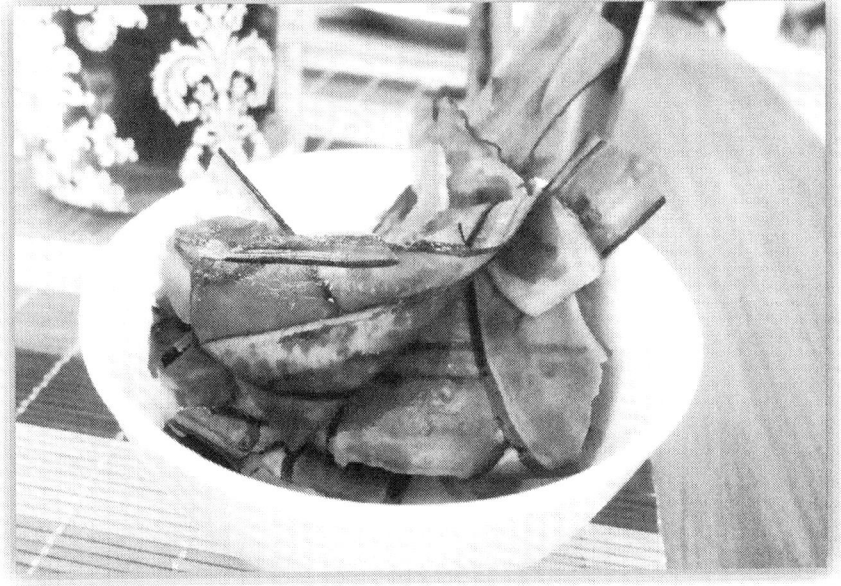

Preparation Time: 5 Minutes
Cooking Time: 10 Minutes
Serving Size: 4

Ingredients:

- 1 Zucchini
- 1 tbsp. Taco Seasoning
- Coconut Oil, as needed

Method of Preparation

- Start by cutting the zucchini into thin strips with the help of a mandolin.
- Next, place these slices on a colander and then generously sprinkle salt over it.
- Allow it to sit for 5 minutes.
- Now, heat the oven to 350 ° F or 175 ° C.
- After that, bake them for 4 to 5 minutes or until it is golden brown colored.
- Finally, sprinkle the taco seasoning over the baked chips and toss well.

Tip: If desired, you can also fry them instead of baking.

Nutritional Information per serving:

✓ Calories: 66Kcal
✓ Fat: 6.9g
✓ Carbohydrates: 1.6g
✓ Proteins: 0.6g
✓ Sodium: 102mg

Prosciutto Wrapped Asparagus

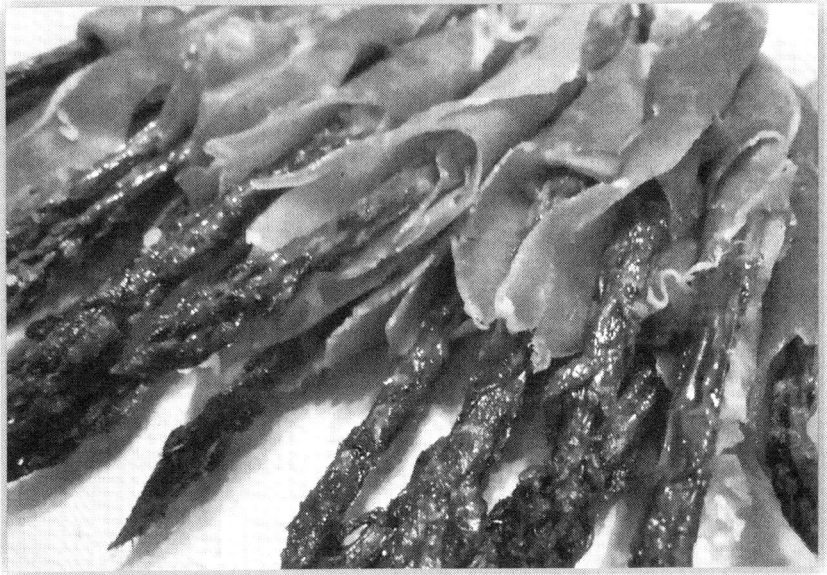

Preparation Time: 10 Minutes
Cooking Time: 15 Minutes
Serving Size: 6

Ingredients:

- 4 tbsp. Almond Meal
- 12 Asparagus Spears
- 2 tbsp. Heavy Cream
- 6 Prosciutto slices, thin
- 4 tbsp. Parmesan, grated

Method of Preparation

- To begin with, discard the ends of the asparagus spears and then place them on a saucepan half-filled with the water.
- Once the water starts boiling, boil the asparagus for 2 to 3 minutes or until it is slightly crunchy. Drain away the water.
- Next, keep the prosciutto slices on the board and place two asparagus diagonally on top.
- After that, mix parmesan and almond meal in another bowl until combined well.
- Now, sprinkle this cheese-almond mixture over the asparagus and drizzle it with heavy cream.
- Roll them up and arrange them on a baking dish.
- Finally, top them with the remaining parmesan almond mixture and bake them for 350 ° F or 175 ° C for 13 minutes or until it is golden in color.

Tip: Instead of an almond meal, you can also use almond flour.

Nutritional Information per serving:

- ✓ Calories: 80Kcal
- ✓ Fat: 5.9g
- ✓ Carbohydrates: 1.7g
- ✓ Proteins: 4.9g
- ✓ Sodium: 170mg

Blueberry Bread

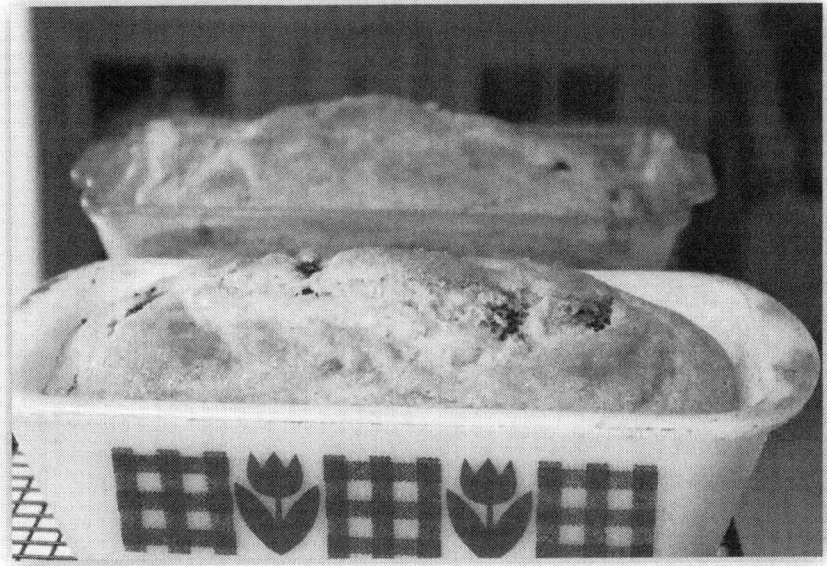

Preparation Time: 15 Minutes
Cooking Time: 50 Minutes
Serving Size: 12

Ingredients:

- ½ cup Almond Flour
- ½ cup Blueberries
- ½ tsp. Salt
- 5 Eggs, preferably farm-raised, large & lightly beaten
- 2 tsp. Baking Powder
- ½ cup Almond Butter
- ½ cup Almond Milk, unsweetened
- ¼ cup Ghee

Method of Preparation

- Preheat the oven to 350 °F.
- After that, melt almond butter and ghee for 30 seconds in a microwave-safe bowl.
- Next, combine almond flour, baking powder, and salt in another bowl and mix well.
- To this, then spoon in the melted nut butter and stir until they are no lumps.
- Whisk the eggs milk in a bowl and set it aside.
- Now, spoon in the blueberries and add them to the batter gradually.
- Line the loaf pan with baking paper and grease it with butter.
- Pour the blueberries batter into the loaf pan and bake for 45 to 50 minutes. Insert a skewer inserted in the center comes clean.
- Allow the loaf to cool for 30 minutes and then serve.
- If desired, toast before serving as it taste best when toasted.

Tip: Instead of almond butter, you can also use cashew butter.

Nutritional Information per serving: (1 serving is one slice)
- ✓ Calories: 156Kcal
- ✓ Fat: 13g
- ✓ Carbohydrates: 3g
- ✓ Proteins: 5g
- ✓ Sodium: 171mg

Conclusion

Diabetic snacks are the perfect solution for you when you would like to spread out your meals for the day in a healthy manner as they help to avoid sugar spikes. Diabetic snacks not only take care of your health but also your cravings to enjoy delicious foods.

This book aims at educating readers about diabetics and healthy diabetic snacks. Dedicated efforts have been made in the book to provide its readers with healthy diabetic snack recipes that they can prepare at home anytime they want and enjoy them guilt-free.

We thank you all for giving their precious time to read this book. We sincerely hope that the recipes covered in the book will inspire its readers to start eating healthy foods. Start your journey by making your first diabetic snack from this book, and continue enjoying the crispy, savory treats.

Thank you all again; good luck.

Printed in Great Britain
by Amazon

44648477R00054